Reflective Practice

A Guide for Nurses and Midwives

Reflective Practice

A Guide for Nurses and Midwives

Beverley J. Taylor

Open University Press
Maidenhead

Open University Press
McGraw–Hill Education
McGraw–Hill House
Shoppenhangers Road
Maidenhead
Berkshire
SL6 2QL

email: enquiries@openup.co.uk
world wide web: www.openup.co.uk

First published in 2000
Reprinted 2001 (twice), 2003, 2004

A catalogue record for this book is available from the British Library.

ISBN 0 335 20689 1 (pb)   0 335 20690 5 (hb)

Library of Congress Cataloging-in-Publication Data
Taylor, Beverley J.
Reflective practice : a guide for nurses and midwives / Beverley J. Taylor.
    p. cm.
Includes bibliographical references and index.
ISBN 0–335–20689–1 (pbk.) – ISBN 0–335–20690–5 (hc.)
1. Nursing–Study and teaching. 2. Nursing–Philosophy. 3.
Midwives–Study and teaching. 2. Self-evaluation. I. Title.
RT73.T29 2000
610.73'01–dc21   00–023298

Printed and bound in Great Britain by Biddles Ltd, King's Lynn, Norfolk

Contents

CONTENTS

Preface

If we have not met already, let me introduce myself. My name is Bev Taylor and I was born in 1951 in Burnie, Tasmania. I was always a thoughtful kind of child, spending a lot of time in my own imagination, making up stories and talking to my cat, 'Tom'. I remember contemplating infinity at the age of seven, pondering space beyond space beyond space. I was also intrigued with parables and metaphors I learned in Sunday School, and I think it is from these beginnings that I have developed my love of words and language. I come from a family of storytellers, the most significant of whom was my father, who wove each story with craft and precision, never exaggerating, but always being true to the events and moods of the story.

My interest in nursing, midwifery and reflection has spanned many years. I have been registered as a nurse since 1971 and as a midwife since 1974. However, even though I have practised, taught and researched midwifery, most of my experience has been in nursing. I became interested in reflective practice when I was studying externally for a Master of Education degree through the School of Education at Deakin University, Geelong in 1987. I was fortunate to be given guidance by Stephen Kemmis, John Smyth and Annette Street, all of whom have remained influential on the ways I view and practise reflection.

However, I suspect that even though the rhetoric has been that there is value in reflective practice for nurses and midwives, the actual practice of it has been done partially, or not at all. What really happens is some token attention to reflection through a few entries in journals for as long as necessary—for example, the length of the clinical placement or the duration of the academic assignment. From what I have seen, reflective practice has become so familiar that it has not been treated seriously by the majority of practitioners who have tried to use it. This is not necessarily a criticism of practitioners; I believe that in many cases they have not been prepared adequately to reflect effectively. I make this claim having seen many units of instruction with reflective practice content. While many of the ideas are in place, I believe that there is relatively little guidance in how to do reflection in a practical and sustained way. Also, some instruction has become bogged down in dense theory which does not always appeal to practitioners, who need to know what to do, why, when and how without developing a treatise on theory and politics. For these reasons, I have written this book in a reader-friendly style, to provide a practical guide for nurses and midwives.

As you read the book, you will notice that I speak directly with you. I have also used first-person pronouns when referring to myself, so that you can develop a sense of having a guide go with you on your reflective journey. Also, in Chapter 2 I introduce two midwives and one nurse, all of whom are currently in practice. Carol, Esther and Michael agreed graciously to use the processes outlined in this book, and to share some of their stories with you.

The main theme of this book is reflection as it applies to the practice of nursing and midwifery. In order to make this handbook as practical as possible, I have included 'reflectors' throughout each chapter. A reflector is the means by which an image is thrown back, such as in a mirror. I use reflectors as means of causing you to reflect on many of the ideas and issues that come up as you progress. I suggest that you buy a fixed-page exercise book, and that you attempt to write notes in response to the reflector items. Write the date and time at the start of each reflection, so that you can return to your ideas and track their evolution over time.

In Chapter 1, I introduce the nature of reflection and suggest that it is based on life and the two main human interests in being and knowing. At the outset, it seems reasonable to think about what reflection is and why it is necessary for human existence. Knowing how to reflect is a process for making sense out of all life experiences. If it is important for people in general ways, reflection is also important for nurses and midwives in specific ways. I define reflection and suggest that it can occur in many ways for purposes such as technical, practical and emancipatory, which are categorised according to the kind of knowledge they involve and the work interests they represent. I suggest that there are many sources of reflection within human life, and that there is value in reflecting. I describe critical thinking as a means of making informed decisions through rationality and link it to technical reflection. In conclusion, I suggest that other ways of knowing and reflecting are worthy of your attention, such as intuitive grasps, creative expression, contemplation and meditation.

In Chapter 2 I introduce two midwives and one nurse, who have adopted the pseudonyms of Carol, Esther and Michael respectively. All of these people are engaged in practice on a regular basis. I describe the nature of nursing and midwifery practice and position it in terms of the nature of bureaucratic work settings, work constraints and daily habits and routines. I suggest that clinicians face many issues in their work settings to demonstrate how and why nursing and midwifery are complex occupations requiring careful attention and reflection.

In Chapter 3 I describe the basic essentials you will need for getting ready to reflect, and liken this phase to preparing for a journey into reflective territories. This chapter gives you some more information about reflective practice, and supplies you with a kitbag of strategies to help you on your way. I also suggest that you have need for determination, courage, a sense of humour and a critical friend, who will help you on your journey by drawing your attention to points of interest along the way so that you can appreciate them more.

In Chapter 4 Esther, Michael and Carol share their reflections on their personal histories, to show the influences of the 'rules of living' that guide their lives as individuals and affect the way they practise at work.

In Chapter 5 I review some literature on professions and professionals and tell you why I think reflection is valuable for all practitioners, and why it is especially valuable for nurses and midwives. To do this, I give my views on the value of nurses and midwives as people and practitioners, and the immense contributions that nursing and midwifery have made, and are continuing to make, to the health of the people in their care. I discuss the value of being a reflective practitioner and learning to value yourself as a person and as a nurse or midwife. Part of this process is about learning to be alert to your practice, to make things better for yourself, other people, the organisation in which you work and your practice discipline. Given that this may sound altogether too much like hard work, I conclude this chapter by looking at some frequently used excuses to avoid reflective practice and some remedies for thinking differently about yourself and taking steps towards becoming a reflective practitioner.

Reflection can be used for many purposes, depending on how and when it is done, by whom and why. In Chapter 6 I introduce three main types of reflection nurses and midwives can use in their work lives, and adapt to their personal lives if they wish. As the basis for understanding how knowledge is related to reflection, I then introduce some nursing and midwifery authors who have categorised ways of knowing. After that I describe empirical, interpretive and critical knowledge and Habermas's 'knowledge-constitutive interests' so you can see how they relate to the kinds of reflection highlighted in this book. Finally, I introduce technical, practical and emancipatory reflection and highlight their relative merits, so you can decide on which type or combination of types of reflection to use for your practice issues.

In Chapter 7 I explain some of the reasons why this process is used for specific purposes and why it creates different outcomes in terms of knowledge of and practical answers to clinical problems. To do this, I step you through the relationship between empirical knowledge and the scientific method, and examine how the process for technical reflection fits with these ideas. I describe the connections between technical reflection and evidence-based practice and suggest that the two processes are highly complementary. The chapter provides an exercise in technical reflection and gives an example of how it has been used by a reflective practitioner.

Sometimes your reflection will be about your own personal and professional growth issues, the nature of phenomena such as the experience of illness, the meaning of events of clinical importance and the dynamics and significance of interpersonal relationships. Practical reflective processes will help you to interpret the communicative aspect of your work setting and the people within it. In Chapter 8 I review some of the assumptions on which practical reflection is based, before I guide you through some reflective exercises and present some stories from Carol's experience.

In Chapter 9 I discuss the third form of reflection, which has the potential to create transformative action. When you want to go beyond prediction provided by technical reflection, and description offered by practical reflection, it might be time to take a more critical view of your practice and the constraints within it by using emancipatory reflection. In this chapter, I review some assumptions underlying emancipatory reflection, before guiding you through the reflective processes and presenting and analysing one of Esther's stories to show you how nurses and midwives can transform their practice using these processes.

I have found that nurses and midwives love to tell and hear stories, and with this in mind, in Chapter 10 I provide you with opportunities to read further practice stories from Esther, Michael and Carol. Through sharing their stories with you, these clinicians offer you a means to improve your reflective skills and knowledge. You can analyse their stories to locate their practice approaches, issues and themes, and as you provide your commentary to them as a critical friend, you may be able to learn from their experiences.

In the final chapter I discuss maintaining your reflective practitioner mentality and the value of finding support systems to keep you on track. This may lead on to organising professional development seminars in your work setting in which to share your experiences, or getting involved in research. In conclusion, this book ends on a positive note as you contemplate the potential of embodying reflective practice in your everyday life and work.

My hopes for the book are that it will provide a practical guide for any nurse or midwife who wants to become a reflective practitioner. I also hope that your reflections allow you to gain deeper insights into your personal life, so that you grow as a person as well as a practitioner. My hopes for nursing and midwifery in the new millennium are that these disciplines will prosper and that practitioners will continue to improve their practices through reflective processes such as those described in this book.

1

The nature of reflection

INTRODUCTION

Life is the basis of reflection, and without it there appears to be no discernible basis for being and knowing. This is not to say that all living things are capable of reflection. The difference between humans and other living entities is the margin between reflective consciousness and awareness. Whereas some forms of communication are possible within some living species in that they have instinctual drives and ways of transmitting their needs, they do not appear to have systematic language and the ability to communicate about communication. As far as can be demonstrated, humans hold the monopoly on thought and reasoned choices, putting them in a responsible position in relation to the other non-thinking living and inanimate entities and phenomena inhabiting and comprising this planet. Thus the ability to think, reason and reflect gives humans awesome privileges and responsibilities for the very integrity of the world itself, a point which may be overlooked by people who consider that everything on earth exists for their use and domination. This idea alone gives humans incredible scope for reflection and informed action.

The objects of reflection are situated in the physical world and in parts of the universe that have been discovered and imagined. Broad and confined areas of inquiry make up a

1

seemingly endless supply of sources of reflection, from 'macro' and 'micro' perspectives, including people as individuals and groups, and places and phenomena above and below the earth, sky and seas within the range of known space. Whatever has been known or can be known is the source of reflection. This means that reflection is an immense project taking up the interest of generations of people, and constituting all of recorded and remembered history. A view of reflection in terms of these proportions makes it so large and complex as to be almost unimaginable and unmanageable, but that is not the intention of this book.

In this chapter I introduce the nature of reflection and suggest that it is based on life and the two main human interests in being and knowing. At the outset, it seems reasonable to think about what reflection is and why it is necessary for human existence. Knowing how to reflect is a process for making sense out of all life experiences. If it is important for people in general ways, reflection is also important for nurses and midwives in specific ways.

I define reflection and suggest that it can occur in many ways for purposes such as technical, practical and emancipatory, which are categorised according to the kind of knowledge they involve and the work interests they represent. I suggest that there are many sources of reflection within human life, and that there is value in reflecting. I describe critical thinking as a means of making informed decisions through rationality and link it to technical reflection. In conclusion, I suggest that other ways of knowing and reflecting are worthy of your attention, such as intuitive grasps, creative expression, contemplation and meditation.

As you will be responding to reflectors throughout the book, I suggest that you record your insights in a fixed-page journal. You will notice many instances throughout the book where I use reflectors to spark reflection and I suggest that you write your responses in your journal. Even though I describe ways of reflecting other than writing, the written word is a mainstay of reflective processes and a journal can serve as a central repository for your thoughts and ideas. So if you do not have an exercise book in which to write, buy one soon and you will have a very important aid for effective reflection. Write the date and time at the start of each reflection, so that you can return to your ideas and track their evolution over time.

DEFINING REFLECTION

In the physical phenomenon sense of the word, to reflect means to throw back from a surface. The most general meaning of reflection is throwing back rays such as heat, sound or light (*Concise English Dictionary* 1984). In the sense in which it is used in this book, reflection means the throwing back of thoughts and memories, in cognitive acts such as thinking, contemplation, meditation and any other form of attentive consideration, in order to make sense of them, and to make contextually appropriate changes if they are required. This definition allows for a wide variety of thinking as the basis for reflection, but it is similar to many other explanations (Mezirow 1981; Boyd and Fales 1983; Boud et al. 1985; Street 1992) due to the inclusion of the two main aspects of thinking as a rational and intuitive process which allows the potential for change.

Schön (1987) differentiated between *reflection-in-action* and *reflection-on-action*. The former occurs during practice when the attentive practitioner watches, interacts and adjusts reactions and approaches through thinking in a focused way while working. There is some debate as to whether reflection-in-action is really possible, given the need to act quickly in complex situations (Clinton 1998); however, it is possible to develop an active participant/thinking observer approach to work, even though it is undoubtedly a complex task. Reflection-on-action occurs after the action when details are recalled through rich description and analysed through careful unpicking and reconstructing of all the aspects of the situation, to gain fresh insights and make amendments if necessary. Although memory may fade with time, it is possible to make sense of work events long after they have happened.

Reflection can occur in many ways for different purposes and this book suggests three main kinds of reflection: technical, practical and emancipatory. They are categorised according to the kind of knowledge they involve and the work interests they represent. Regardless of the kind, and irrespective of the reasons for which they are used, forms of reflection provide

3

processes whereby everyday events of life can be looked at carefully and sorted through systematically for their patterns, issues, instructive value and potential modification.

Technical reflection, based on the scientific method and rational, deductive thinking, will allow you to generate and validate empirical knowledge through rigorous means, so that you can be assured that work procedures are based on scientific reasoning. *Practical reflection* leads to interpretation for description and explanation of human interaction in social existence. *Emancipatory reflection* leads to 'transformative action' which seeks to free nurses and midwives from taken-for-granted assumptions and oppressive forces which limit them and their practice. All kinds of knowledge can be generated through reflection and nurses and midwives can benefit from a range of reflective processes.

Think about what reflection means to you. You might like to look up definitions in several dictionaries, or discuss the meaning of the term with your friends. Jot down some ideas in a journal, or speak them into an audiomachine, until you have your own definition of reflection.

To what extent does your definition agree with mine, or those offered by the authors cited in this section?

Keep a record of your thoughts on the meaning of reflection and refer back to it as often as you like, to see if your definition needs amendment as you progress though this handbook.

SOURCES OF REFLECTION

Life is a source of reflection. In this section I elaborate on this thought, to show how central and all-inclusive reflection is to human existence. Although it is not intended to be an exhaustive list of possible sources of reflection, I refer to general patterns of daily life, work, art and religion, which are some of the fundamental interests on which people may choose to reflect. My reason for doing this is to show that everything of interest to human life is a potential source of reflection.

Life as source of reflection

Life is a rich area for reflection. Human life is about day-to-day existence and the choices people make in relation to their lives and other people and events. As sentient beings, humans have the capacity to make sense of their lives and to learn from their challenges and triumphs. Whether engaged in searching for meaning in their own lives, or finding the answers to difficult questions external to them, the potential is enormous for reflection on a number of fronts.

One of the biggest pursuits in the course of my life has been the search for the reasons why I am living at all. I might spend my whole life earning a living, building relationships, contributing to society and being a good citizen, but the underlying reason for being here may be to find out the meaning of my life. The big questions for me ultimately become: 'Why am I here?' 'What is the meaning of life?' This type of questioning is what philosophers do to some extent, because they search for the meaning of human life as it relates to existence and for what counts as knowledge and truth. On an individual level, however, the inquiry may be more about making sense out of the everyday events and issues that act as catalysts for self-awareness and personal growth.

If you listen carefully, you may find that people's views about life are often coloured by some overriding personal perspective, such as their political persuasion, religious beliefs, gender, group affiliations and so on. For example, in referring to Karl Marx, Friedrich Engels (in Seldes 1983: 242), a German socialist and associate of Marx, said: 'He discovered the simple fact (heretofore hidden beneath ideological excrescences) that human beings must have food and drink, clothing and shelter, first of all before they can interest themselves in politics, art, religion, and the like.' Engels was referring to the responsibility of the state to provide basic essentials for people, so that they could aspire to higher ideals. It is interesting to note that, in spite of all his influence in political thought, Marx took a practical view and prioritised basic human needs for food and shelter above the needs for reflection and intellectual pursuits.

Oscar Wilde (in Seldes 1983: 744), an English writer, gave his view of life when he said: 'The only thing that one really knows about human nature is that it changes. Change is the one quality we can predicate on it. The systems that fail are

5

those that rely on the permanency of human nature, and not on its growth and development.' Wilde critiqued issues of life as an artist and he acknowledged the influence of art in setting trends and changing people's perspectives on taken-for-granted social norms.

Life offers humans a series of lessons if they are open to learning them. Whether the lessons have to do with loss and grief, or gains and joys, life events are potentially instructive as people attempt to make sense of them. Life events such as death, separation, illness and accidents may act as catalysts for deep inner reflection, which reaches to some fundamental 'bottom lines' about what life is about and whether it is worth living at all. Interestingly, gains and joys such as births, marriages and health, as well as routine, unaffected existence, do not seem to have the same impact for deep personal reflection as gut-wrenching tragedies such as sudden, unexpected death. Even though they may be appreciated for their positive value, gains and joys seem to be taken on without much deliberation and added to life's repertoire of events in a grateful, yet unexamined way. It is possible to learn through gain and joy, yet it seems to me that the events which 'pull us up in our tracks' are the ones which hurt us in some way and force us to make sense of our wounds.

Daily human life varies according to where it is being played out, why and when, but it has certain common features, such as those outlined by Maslow (1970). This celebrated but dated work is still as relevant as when Abraham Maslow put it forward for comment. It never ceases to impress me that the 'obvious' and simplest statements about life can affect me most deeply. It makes good sense to me to agree with Maslow that I need to have my basic physiological and safety needs met first, before I can begin to think of satisfying my higher order needs for love, self-esteem and self-actualisation.

Life can go on day after day, and it may seem like nothing more than a series of events if it is not considered carefully for its instructive value. Rituals, symbols, habits and routines can become so enmeshed in daily life that, even though they may be heavy with meaning, they may be enacted in a seemingly flippant and thoughtless way. For example, a family may interact in complex ways with each person appearing to know the others' idiosyncrasies, and family cohesion is not really tested until arguments arise from contradictory interpretations of what is happening, why and how, to whom, at any given time. Similarly, a group of people may be in consensus as to the meaning they assign to their rituals, symbols, habits and routines, while other people may be totally unaware of their significance. For example, in certain cultures, the left hand is reserved to clean up after body functions and the right hand only is used for eating. You can look 'out of place' and ignorant by contravening this practice.

The whole world is made up by collections of people who have developed their own language-based cultures over time with little or no relation to the beliefs, rituals, symbols and practices of other groups of people living in different locations. The diversity of how people live their daily lives makes up the rich complexity of our multicultural world. In a general sense, therefore, if impressions are not checked within and between individuals and groups for the negotiated meaning of rituals, symbols, habits and routines, interpretations can be varied, and confusion, disapproval and conflict can arise. Reflection is the key to making sense of different human practices and to making contextually appropriate changes to them if they are required.

Have you ever mused on the meaning of life?
When was it?
What did you conclude?
Have your thoughts on the meaning of life changed over time?
If you have not mused on the meaning of life, why not try now?
Write some ideas in a journal. Try to use sentences which describe as clearly and richly as possible the ways in which you are thinking about life as a source of reflection.

Work as source of reflection

Unpaid and paid work are part of life. Work hours take up a great deal of time, and their content and processes can pass by aimlessly and insignificantly if not analysed carefully to make sense of them. In other words, work becomes a set of tasks which pay the bills or fill in idle time if they are not considered for their intrinsic worth. People invest themselves in work activities and bring to public work settings parts of their private identities. Work involves rituals, habits and routines that keep actions focused and relevant. While these work activities serve specific purposes, their inherent meaning may be rendered invisible by their constancy and familiarity, so that they remain unconsidered and insignificant. Work time is admitted by thinking people into life events which are worthy of reflection, given that paid and unpaid work plays such an important role in people's lives and it is one way through which humans come to define themselves.

Reflection in and on nursing practice is necessary to alert clinicians to the intricacies of nursing practice and the knowledge embedded in it. Nursing is situated in the everyday life of its participants, and the familiarity of the total context can cause nurses to take for granted those events and activities which give nursing its essential qualities. Just as one's personal life can become an unconsidered stream of events, so also can work experiences.

How do you react to the idea that work is a source of reflection?

Do you agree or disagree? Why?

Talk to work colleagues about this idea and find out what they think.

Art as a source of reflection

Art reflects life through many representations. Painters, poets, sculptors, potters, dancers, actors, musicians and others around the world and throughout time have interpreted their views of life through artistic practices. All of life is rich as a potential source of inspiration, including people and their relationships to other people, living entities, nature, places, time past, present and future, and phenomena of all kinds. The quest to know the nature of oneself through reflection and personal ruminations has been described in literature and all forms of art are rich sources of reflection. Art is at the same time the product and the generator of reflection and its impact is immense on the traditions of reflective consciousness of humans throughout the world.

Think about whether any form of art has been a source of reflection for you.
What was it?
How did it affect you?
Why did it affect you?

Religious teachings as sources of reflection

Reflection has been enshrined in human activity through the sacred texts and teachings of various religions. Through religious practices, humans reflect on the nature of human life and its connections with higher consciousness. Reflection takes on various forms in spiritual life, such as reading and thinking about sacred writings, the performance of ceremonies and rituals, prayer, meditation, contemplation, singing songs of praise, storytelling and inspirational writing.

Each religion guides its followers in specific fundamental principles about life and sacred entities and ideals. The Bible suggests that humans think on things of a positive and pure nature. The Bhagavad Gita of the Hindu faith finds stillness in reflection through meditation; Buddha's teachings resulted from deep meditation and reflection.

The sacred teachings of indigenous peoples are not often written in books. For example, Indigenous Australians transmit their religious reflections through stories, ceremonies and private meetings. Reflection on spiritual matters is at the level of the earth and sky and on the beings of the Dreaming. Thus, for Indigenous Australians, all of Nature is subject to reflection and honour. The creator god withdraws to the distant heavens where he/she cannot be reached by human beings, and is not consulted for everyday events. Only for the most sacred initiations will the god be present. These beliefs and others form the core of religious practices and give a focus for reflection on people's place in relation to the land and natural elements.

The need to reflect on forms of higher consciousness has been enshrined in human activity, through the sacred texts and teachings of various religions. Practised in many forms and

9

with many different kinds of gods and godesses, the act of reflection on sacred teachings and texts provides a rich source for people trying to make sense of their earthly existence.

> To what extent do religious and spiritual teachings and practices influence you as sources of reflection in your life?
>
> Are there any particular religious or spiritual principles or practices which are foundational to the ways you live your life and practice as a nurse or midwife?
>
> Write some responses to these questions in your journal.

THE VALUE OF REFLECTION

Judgments are made as to what is valuable in life. One definition of 'valuable' refers to the worth, utility and importance of someone or something. Therefore, it follows that when something is deemed valuable it is precious and worthy. Reflection is a valuable part of human life. There is value in reflection as it turns an unconsidered life into one which is consciously aware, self-potentiating and purposeful. Plato went so far as to say that 'The unreflected life is not worth living'. Imagine going through life without a second thought as to what has happened, when, where, why, how, to whom or what, and with what consequences. Memories would be foggy, and stories would be without purpose, morals and messages. Historical accounts, if recorded, would be confused and unsubstantiated. People's actions would be devoid of judgments and consequences. There would be no basis for personal and collective growth. It is difficult for me to imagine an unreflected life of this planet and its people. Can you?

Reflection becomes the basis for history. Unless events in time are analysed for their instructive worth, nothing can be learned from them. It is reasonable to assume that if people do not consider the events of their past, they are powerless to shape their future, because they will not have taken advantage of the lessons that can be learned through frank appraisal of

10

group and individual experiences. However, even with all its positive attributes, reflection is not a panacea for all the world's ills. Sadly—or perhaps inevitably—even with reflection on history, major negative world phenomena still occur, such as wars, prejudice, greed, famine, crimes against humanity and inequalities of many kinds.

This book places a positive light on the value of reflection, based on its potential for making sense of experiences and phenomena and making changes in future cases if that is appropriate. Nurses and midwives are kept busy in their daily work. If they are convinced of the value of reflection for their life generally, and their work specifically, they will make time to practise reflective thinking for their professional and personal benefit.

CRITICAL THINKING AND REFLECTION

The ability to think in a systematic and rational way separates humans from other species and gives people reflective consciousness. Thinking is integral to reflection, and the kind of thinking required for making sense of personal and work events can differ according to the demands of the situation and the enormity of the task. For example, searching for answers to difficult questions about quantum physics is a different cognitive task and uses complex thinking processes, relative to deciding what to wear to a concert, or when to get out of bed in the morning.

When thinking takes on complex proportions, it takes on a more critical nature. Authors (e.g. Bandman and Bandman 1995; van Hooft et al. 1995) have described critical thinking and emphasised its use in nursing and midwifery. All of these authors agree that critical thinking is essential for safe practice and that rationality is its first requirement. In this section, I explain what critical thinking is, what it comprises, the skills and attitudes required to do it successfully, and how this all relates to reflection.

Definitions of critical thinking

According to Bandman and Bandman (1995: 7) critical thinking is 'the rational examination of ideas, inferences, assumptions, principles, arguments, conclusions, issues, statements, beliefs,

11

and actions'. They clarify their definition by stating that critical thinking includes scientific reasoning, the use of the nursing process, decision-making and reasoning about issues. Adding further specifications to the definition, they make it clear that critical thinking is:

> reasoning in which we analyse the use of language, formulate problems, clarify and explicate assumptions, weigh evidence, evaluate conclusions, discriminate between good and bad arguments, and seek to justify those facts that result in credible beliefs and actions.

Van Hooft et al. (1995: 6–7) are keen to define the first important element of critical thinking as rational thinking. In supporting their prioritisation, they use the Bandman and Bandman (1995) definition, but they follow this up with some important qualifying statements, which describe the nature of critical thinking and of critical thinkers. They summarise critical thinking as being rational, practical as well as theoretical, and conducive to dialogue, and describe critical thinkers as committed, self-aware and sympathetic to the commitments of others. This adds some human aspects to the definition of critical thinking, which are missing from Bandman and Bandman's definition. These authors tend to feature rationality as an objective process, and to understate the subjective qualities of the people possessing the capacity for rational thought.

Wilkinson (1996: 26) defines critical thinking as 'both an attitude and a reasoning process involving a number of intellectual skills' and places rationality at the head of the list of characteristics. Interestingly, Wilkinson's account of critical thinking has the strongest human emotion content in that, while she acknowledges the central role of rationality, she also emphasises the subjective side of critical thinking, by describing the skills and attitudes of critical thinkers.

Component parts

Whereas the definitions of critical thinking may be useful in their comprehensiveness, they introduce many words which require definition. Before moving on to look at the skills and attitudes required for critical thinking, I will clarify some words, such as reasoning, scientific reasoning, assumptions and arguments.

Reasoning refers to the act of drawing conclusions from *premises*, which are statements leading up to end findings or summary statements. Premises show a discernible pattern of thought which follows logically from a former idea. For example, reasoning often includes 'if–then' statements, such as: 'If nurses work on improving their own patterns of communication, then they will be better able to develop therapeutic relationships with patients'. Reasoning may have many steps in the pathway between the original and end statements. The more complex the reasoning, the greater the need for more premises or propositions to make and support a stronger argument.

In this context, an *argument* is not a quarrel; rather, it means a well thought out and delivered defence of a point of view supported by sound reasoning. Not all premises in an argument may be stated openly—they may be hidden as *assumptions,* which may be discerned as 'gaps' in the logic of arguments. It is not difficult to recognise assumptions in an argument because people tend to make them frequently, in the often-mistaken belief that others will be able to 'fill in the gaps' through their own knowledge and experience of the area being discussed.

Words such as because, hence, since, so, therefore and thus may be used to maintain the flow of the argument and indicate the connections between the ideas expressed in the statements used to support the conclusions. For example, reasoning may be presented thus:

> Communication is an important interpersonal skill, which all people need, because it is integral to everyday life. Since nurses care for people who may not be able to express their needs, it is especially important for nurses to refine their communication skills; therefore, professional development sessions should include opportunities to improve knowledge and practice of communication skills.

Scientific reasoning refers to a certain kind of argument which reflects the assumptions underlying 'the scientific model'. The main features of scientific knowledge are that it claims to be objective (free from emotionality), systematic, rigorous in terms of the way in which it is organised and validated, and able to predict and explain relationships between variables. Typically, the scientific approach to reasoning is to state a problem, give a preliminary hypothesis setting out the expected relationships between variables, collect more facts in order to formulate an hypothesis, deduce further consequences, test those consequences, and finally apply the findings to confirm or disconfirm the hypothesis (Bandman and Bandman 1995).

This kind of reasoning is advantageous in thinking through the consequences of adaptations to nursing and midwifery procedures, so that they could be made more effective and based on sound scientific reasoning rather than folklore or some other untested assumptions. Scientific reasoning of this kind is structured into quantitative research designs to ensure that methods produce credible and dependable results. As this book cannot deal with all that is inferred by the mention of research, I would like to suggest that you consult some research texts if you would like to pursue these ideas (see Polgar and Thomas 1995; Polit and Hungler 1997; Roberts and Taylor 1998).

Think about work situations in which you need to think critically. Make a list of them. Look carefully at the list and see if critical thinking is needed in certain kinds of situations.

Are there common kinds of situations? If so, what are they like? If not, how do the situations differ?

Why do these situations require critical thinking?

Skills and attitudes

According to Wilkinson (1996), the cognitive skills required for critical thinking include decision making and problem-solving methods. Nurses and midwives make decisions constantly about the best ways of achieving clinical goals. Problem-solving involves assessing, planning, implementing and evaluating the best courses of action in given situations so that the most effective care can be negotiated. Wilkinson suggests that methods of problem-solving might include intuition as described by Benner (1984) and Benner and Tanner (1987), the scientific method and the nursing process. Intuition is part of expert clinical practice and is acquired through years of knowledge and experience when patterns and cues from prior like instances present rapidly and completely to an expert's consciousness. I have described the scientific method earlier in this chapter, and the nursing process is a well documented problem-solving process which has been used by nurses and midwives for many decades. If you need to explore this method further, I suggest you read Wilkinson (1996), because she explores the nursing process through a critical thinking approach.

The attitudes suggested for critical thinking include thinking independently, intellectual humility, courage, empathy, integrity and perseverance. Wilkinson (1996: 29–32) also suggests that other attitudes required are faith in reason, fairmindedness and the need to explore thoughts and feelings. Not surprisingly, independent thinking requires critical thinkers to be able to think and to 'stand up' for themselves. Nurses and midwives must be able to be autonomous, because so many work decisions must be made quickly for the best results. Intellectual humility means being prepared to own up to what you do not know, so that you do not act self-deceptively. Intellectual courage is needed when critical thinkers are prepared to reassess their own ideas in the face of new information which is based on sound reason and evidence. Intellectual empathy is the ability to imagine yourself 'in the place of others in order to understand them and their actions and beliefs' (1996: 30). Intellectual integrity is about being honest and consistent in your thinking. Intellectual perseverance is about being determined to sort through issues and options to overcome confusion and complexities. Faith in reason refers to a belief in the soundness of rationality and it allows critical thinkers 'to distinguish intuition from prejudice' (1996: 31). Fairmindedness occurs when critical thinkers 'consider opposing points of view and listen with an open mind to new ideas' (1996: 31). Finally, Wilkinson (1996: 31–32) suggests that 'all feelings are based on some kind of thinking, and all thought creates some kind of feeling'. Knowing this, critical thinkers consider their own and the other person's feelings, in order to appreciate the behaviour being enacted.

Although van Hooft et al. (1995) deal extensively with the intellectual skills needed for critical thinking, they also make it clear that 'critical thinking does not consist only of rational cleverness. It includes empathy and sensitive perception.' (1995: 5) Maintaining dogged attention to the need for rationality,

Bandman and Bandman (1995: 7–8) do not describe the skills and attitudes of the critical thinker as such; rather, they provide a checklist of the functions critical thinkers should perform. They suggest that critical thinkers:

- use the process of critical thinking in all of daily living;
- discriminate among the uses and misuses of language in nursing;
- identify and formulate nursing problems;
- analyse meanings of terms in relation to their indication, their cause or purpose and their significance;
- analyse arguments and issues into premises and conclusions;
- examine nursing assumptions;
- report data and clues accurately;
- make and check inferences based on data, making sure that the inferences are at least plausible;
- formulate and clarify beliefs;
- verify, corroborate and justify claims, beliefs, conclusions, decisions and actions;
- give relevant reasons for beliefs and conclusions;
- formulate and clarify value judgments;
- evaluate the soundness of conclusions.

Review the various skills and attitudes connected with critical thinking.

Which of these skills and attitudes do you think you possess?

To help you to reflect on your critical thinking skills and attitudes, think of a situation in which you needed to use reasoning of this nature.

In your journal, write responses to these questions:

- What was the nature of the problem?
- Where did it happen?
- When did it happen?
- Who was involved?
- How were you involved?
- Why was critical thinking necessary?

How were you able to assist through critical thinking? Write an outline of your reasoning process. How did you help? In other words, what were the outcomes of your intervention through critical thinking?

Keep a record of this reflection, because it will be very useful combined with other responses to reflectors in this handbook.

The relation of critical thinking to reflection

Reflection requires thinking of some kind. I have already defined reflection as the throwing back of thoughts and memories, in cognitive acts such as thinking, contemplation, meditation and any other form of attentive consideration, in order to make sense of them, and to make contextually appropriate changes if they are required. In the latter part of this chapter, I have focused on critical thinking as one way of thinking about certain issues in nursing and midwifery. Critical thinking has been described and endorsed at length by authors convinced of its necessity in making informed clinical decisions based on rationality. There is much more to reasoning than I have overviewed in this chapter—in fact, it is the subject of several books. Two excellent books which give detailed discussions of what is required and how to practise the rationality involved in critical thinking have been cited previously (Bandman and Bandman 1995; van Hooft et al. 1995). Reasoning of this kind is quite complex and it requires your considered attention to do it well.

In this book I make the distinction between technical, practical and emancipatory types of reflection, based on my underlying assumptions that certain kinds of knowledge exist to serve different purposes. Therefore, if knowledge is generated through reflection, the way in which this is done will differ somewhat according to the type of reflective task. I explore this idea fully in Chapter 6; suffice to say at this point that I consider that the kind of reflection for which critical thinking serves the greatest advantage is technical reflection when the need for scientific reasoning is paramount.

As you begin to get involved in reflection, you may not

necessarily ask yourself which kind of thinking you are using to respond to the reflective tasks I set out for you in this book.

The reason for alerting you to critical thinking is to give you more choices about the ways in which you choose to reflect. If you require careful, fully analytical reasoning to assure you of the conclusions you have drawn in relation to some objective issues in your practice, critical thinking processes are worthy of your attention and practice. Whatever you do in reflection, some kind of reasoning will almost invariably be involved, even if it is only to make direct connections between events to find patterns and themes in your work. The reason I make the qualification that reasoning will almost invariably be involved is to leave open other, less acknowledged and supported, options—options that are nevertheless claimed by some people to have real importance in their reflective practices. I refer here to intuitive grasps, creative expression, and inner knowing that is not easily rationalised, such as contemplation and meditation.

Sometimes connections are made between events with what appears to be no conscious effort at thinking. It is as though the answers are already there just as the questions are posed or even a split second before they are articulated. It is possible to get an intuitive grasp such as: 'I've got it! I know!' Some people explain this phenomenon by appealing to the effects of experience, while others claim that it is independent of experience—they would say that *it just is*. Whatever the source of knowing, either through experience or direct awareness, however gained, intuitive grasps can occur and, having happened, are worthy of reflection. The reason for needing to explore intuitive grasps further is that the conclusion thus gained may not turn out to be reliable given the passage of time, circumstances and other information. If intuitive grasps are to be acknowledged—and I consider that they can be—then they can be balanced with further reflection that tries to find some other evidence for the conclusions which have come so rapidly. Time may show that the grasps were groundless, or conversely they may reveal deep knowing of unquestionable value. My suggestion is that they be noticed and explored to see if they can add to the outcomes of reflection. It is too easy to dismiss out of hand things that cannot be explained objectively, but if they are entertained in a tentative way until further information is gained, they might prove to be complementary to methods of thinking based on some form of rationality.

Have you ever experienced an 'intuitive grasp'? That is, have you ever sensed an answer or insight instantaneously, without seeming to go through a systematic thinking process? The following questions may help you to write a story about an 'intuitive grasp'.

Think of an incident either at home or at work, in which you felt you experienced an 'intuitive grasp'.

- What happened?
- Where did it happen?
- When did it happen?
- Who was involved?
- How were you involved?
- Why do you think it was an 'intuitive grasp'?
- Did the passage of time and circumstances show that your 'intuitive grasp' was accurate?
- How do you explain the phenomenon now? That is, do you think that your 'intuitive grasp' was connected with prior experiences, or was it somehow outside everything you have known before?

Reflection can be facilitated through creative expression. Whether the awareness of the expression precedes or follows reflection is a moot point, but that it can occur is sufficient enough to admit it into the ways in which 'thinking' can be done. For example, I may not know where to start in reflecting on how I feel about the death of a patient I have nursed for some time, so I could paint a picture and see what comes out. Alternatively, I could write a poem and let it wander until it tells me how I feel about the death. Maybe I could even allow my body to tell me in a dance I do in private as I think of the person. I could sing a song I create myself, noticing the words I sing and the sound of the music I create. The ways in which I can reflect creatively on anything in my clinical practice and my life are limited only by my imagination and my motivation to try.

Other forms of reflective thinking or inner knowing which cannot easily be rationalised are contemplation and meditation. A lot has been written about these forms of reflecting (Brennan 1987, 1993; Capra 1988, 1992; Houston 1987; Judith 1992) and it is not my intention to go into issues such as their worthiness as methods, or how or why they are done. The contradiction here is that they facilitate reflection by clearing the mind of excess thoughts, making the way clear for focused and uncomplicated reflection. The value of these forms of reflection is in clearing away the debris of too much rationality, so that a different starting point in thinking is reached, allowing different perspectives to be gained. This is in contradiction to other forms of reflection such as those described in this book, which engage you actively in posing and exploring questions about yourself and your practice. None of this will make much sense to you if you have not involved and do not intend to involve yourself in some form of contemplative or meditative practice. This is OK. If it does not strike a chord with you, it is simply not for you. I raise it here for you to consider so you can find out more about it if it strikes you as interesting and admit it to your range of possibilities.

SUMMARY

In this chapter I introduced you to the nature of reflection and suggested that it is based on life and the two main human interests in being and knowing. I defined reflection as the throwing back of thoughts and memories, in cognitive acts such as thinking, contemplation, meditation and any other form of attentive consideration, in order to make sense of them and to make contextually appropriate changes if required. This definition allows for a wide variety of thinking as the basis for reflection, but it is similar to many other previous explanations. I suggested that reflection can occur in many ways for different purposes and this book will describe three main kinds of reflection—technical, practical and emancipatory—categorised according to the kind of knowledge they involve and the work interests they represent.

I suggested that there are many sources of reflection within human life, including unpaid and paid work, art and sacred texts and teachings of various religions. The value of reflection depends on the importance people place on thinking about various aspects of human life. I described critical thinking as a means of making informed decisions through rationality. The kind of reflection for which critical thinking serves the greatest advantage is technical reflection when the need for scientific reasoning is paramount. The reason I alerted you to critical thinking was to give you more choices in the ways you choose to reflect. If you require careful, fully analytical reasoning to assure you of the conclusions you have drawn in relation to some objective issues in your practice, critical thinking processes are worthy of your attention and practice. I suggested that other ways of knowing and reflecting are worthy of your attention, such as intuitive grasps, creative expression, contemplation and meditation.

2

The nature of nursing
and midwifery

The complexity of nursing and midwifery means that it is not a simple job to be an effective clinician. With so many tasks, roles, relationships, expectations and unforseen elements to negotiate, it is no wonder that practice has a tendency to become chaotic and unpredictable. In the relative madness that makes up a work day, the least you might hope for is that your work will be safe and polite, and the very best that it will be therapeutic and genuine. In this book I intend to move you towards the therapeutic and genuine end of the continuum, by helping you to identify and act on those factors that prevent you from being as effective as you might ideally hope to be on a regular basis at work.

In this chapter I introduce you to two midwives and one nurse. All of these people are engaged in practice on a regular basis. Also in this chapter, I describe the nature of nursing and midwifery practice and position it in terms of the nature of bureaucratic work settings, work constraints and daily habits and routines. I describe the issues clinicians face in their work settings to show how and why nursing and midwifery are complex occupations requiring careful attention to many aspects.

I would like to thank the nurses and midwives who offered their help in the writing of this book. These clinicians worked with me by using the processes described in this book to reflect on their practice. It was not always possible for me to follow each story through to its conclusion and apply my full attention as a critical friend. However, in most cases, and with minimal help from me, Carol, Esther and Michael were able to identify problems in their practice, to work towards critiquing the constraints, and to reconstruct their situations. You will find that these personal and practice stories from reflective practitioners appear throughout the book to help you understand the processes. For example, at the end of this chapter, some stories will be related which show the many issues nurses and midwives face as part of their working days.

CAROL

Carol 'went nursing' at Prince Alfred Hospital in Sydney in 1981 when she was 18 years old. She completed her midwifery training at the Royal Hospital for Women, Paddington, and has been practising as a midwife since. She is working presently in the North Island of New Zealand as a midwife and is studying in a Master of Women's Health course. Carol hopes to 'give the control to the women, educate them, and empower them'. She says: 'If I can make even the slightest difference in someone's life, then my practice is worthwhile.'

ESTHER

Esther has had approximately 20 years' experience in nursing and midwifery. She completed her general nurse training in the United Kingdom in 1978 and her midwifery training in Australia in 1985. Esther graduated with Distinction from a Bachelor of Health Science (Nursing) degree in 1991, and she has completed an Advanced Nursing Certificate in Women's Health, and a Graduate Certificate in Advanced Midwifery. Esther practises as a multi-skilled nurse/midwife in a small rural hospital, which she finds 'incredibly challenging' and she says that she has to be 'a jack of all trades, and master of them all, rather than a master of none!' Esther is a Clinical Nurse Specialist in research, particularly midwifery, and she is working currently to promote evidence-based practice and introduce alternative modes of midwifery care in the hospital in which she works.

MICHAEL

Michael has been nursing since he completed his general nurse training in a large rural hospital in Victoria in 1986. Michael worked in orthopaedics and critical care for four years and since then he has nursed people who have orthopaedic high dependency and are recovering from spinal surgery. Michael says that his approach to nursing is 'sharing—making patients part of the decision-making process regarding their care'. He always discusses what he would see as a reasonable plan for the day, but he is happy to negotiate a different plan if it is more suitable to the patient. He loves to listen to patients telling him their stories, taking the time to find out about life outside a hospital room, so that he can piece together the whole picture. However, the major thing he strives for is a sense of fun and enjoyment in his work. He says: 'When a job ceases to be enjoyable I leave to find something else. That's why, after 15 years of nursing, I am nine years away from long service leave.'

NURSING AND MIDWIFERY

Nursing scholars have been so keen to define nursing that a 'science' has sprung up around that very activity. Over the years, so much has been written about the nature and effect of nursing in books, journal articles, conference presentations and research projects that it would need a small library just to track the progress of the literature. Nursing has been described from Nightingale to the present day and many of the definitions vary according to perceptions of the roles, responsibilities and relationships of nurses with patients.

Midwifery is a growing discipline, having struggled in the twentieth century to regain its power and autonomy and to resituate the experiences of women and babies back into a health model of women-centred care. For this reason, there is to date not much theory which is midwifery-exclusive, but midwifery enjoys a very proud history which dates back to

24

well before the time of the 'wisewomen' who were also suspected of being witches. Even though midwifery has been keen to divorce itself from biomedical influences, midwives are willing to share some of nursing's theoretical content, especially those parts which emphasise holism and client-centred care.

Write some responses to these questions:

- Have you ever wondered how you would describe the nature and effects of the work you do if you had to define it in one or two sentences?
- How would you go about defining nursing or midwifery? What is it? What does it do?
- How does your work differ from other non-professional forms of caring which offer nurse-like and midwife-like services?

Nursing

A classic definition of nursing was given by Nightingale (1893 in Seymer 1955: 334–35), who believed that '[nursing puts] us in the best possible conditions for Nature to restore or to preserve health—to prevent or to cure disease or injury'. Frederick and Northam (1938: 3) claimed that 'nursing requires the application of scientific knowledge and nursing skills and affords the opportunities for constructive work in the care and relief of patients and their families'. Peplau (1952: 16) described nursing as 'a significant, therapeutic, interpersonal process'. Henderson (1955: 4) agreed with her contemporaries that 'nursing is primarily assisting the individual (sick or well) in the performance of those activities contributing to health, or its recovery (or to a peaceful death) that he [sic] would perform unaided if he [sic] had the necessary strength, will, or knowledge'.

Orem (1959) and Kinlein (1977) built on the concept of self-care, putting the responsibility back into the hands of the person receiving care, with the nurse giving assistance only as required. Abdellah et al. (1960: 24) claimed:

nursing is a service to individuals and to families; therefore, to society. It is based upon an art and science which mold the attitudes, intellectual competencies, and technical skills of the individual nurse into the desire and ability to help people, sick or well, cope with their health needs, and may be carried out under general or specific medical direction.

Orlando (1961), Rogers (1961) and Wiedenbach (1964) agreed with the supportive role of the nurse depicted by Nightingale, Henderson, Orem, Kinlein and Abdellah et al. Travelbee (1971: 7) viewed nursing as 'an interpersonal process whereby the professional nurse practitioner assists an individual, family, or community to prevent or cope with the experience of illness and suffering and, if necessary, to find meaning in these experiences'.

King (1971: 22) continued the theme of nursing as being supportive in 'a process of action, reaction, interaction, and transaction'. For Roy (1976: 18), nursing was about supporting people's adaptation. Paterson and Zderad (1976: 51) described humanistic nursing as 'the act of nursing, the intersubjective transactional relation, the dialogue experience, lived in concert between persons where comfort and nurturance prod mutual unfolding'. Since the 1980s, nursing has been described in terms of the therapeutic effect of the nurse–patient relationship, but the current trends are towards poststructuralist and postmodern views of nursing, in which the political nature of theory and practice of nursing is emphasised, and in which there is a tendency to let go of grand narratives about what constitutes the 'truth' about nursing (Greenwood 1996; Keleher and McInerney 1998; Kermode and Brown 1996). These and other authors are suggesting that nursing is part of a postmodern world in which ideas are left open to question and no absolute knowledge can be claimed as the theory of nursing.

Which of the previous definitions of nursing best suit your definition?
How and why do they suit your definition?

Nurses

Nurses work with people throughout the various phases of their lives. Through their knowledge and skills, nurses assist in facilitating those conditions in which people are assisted to feel better and/or to die peacefully. Experienced nurses work in seemingly effortless ways to care for people. When the science of the theory and the art of the practice of nursing come together, it can be seen that the work of nursing has great value in creating those conditions in which mothers and others feel 'cared for' by nurses. Nurses are key workers in the health care system, working around the clock to care for people facing illness and loss. Nursing practice is something to be valued for its ability to make a difference in the lives of these people.

Being a nurse is about being busy. Every day there is so much to do, to ensure that all of the work is done in a way that is safe and thorough. Much of work life involves repetition, because each new patient has his or her own particular concerns and nurses need to accommodate these concerns, whilst ensuring that the standard care practices are followed. With so much to do and so much need for repetition, it may come as no surprise that nurses may develop a robot-like approach to much of their work.

Although nurses have been aligned with doctors and the biomedical model, much of nurses' work is unique and rests entirely on nurses for its development and validity. Nurses are responsible for nursing work, and even though in some settings they may still be responsible directly to doctors in carrying out medical regimes, nurses are nevertheless autonomous within the realms of their own practice, having direct and sole authority over all work which is uniquely nursing.

Midwifery

The term 'midwife' means 'a woman who is with the mother at birth' (Oakley and Houd 1990: 17). It is reasonable to imagine that women have been attending other women in birthing since time began. The practice of midwifery continued unaffected until the Middle Ages, when it received negative attention from the male-dominated state and the church, at the time of the witch hunts in Europe which lasted from the fourteenth to seventeenth centuries (McCool and McCool 1989). The midwives of that time worked with herbs and other healing modalities. The first regulation of their practice came about because of fear of their powers as lay healers and their supposed identity as witches, together with the political and religious threat they posed to the dominant forces, by virtue of being self-directed and influential women (Ehrenreich and English 1973; Kitzinger 1991). It is not surprising to find that the extermination of midwives as witches came at a time when medicine was gaining ascendency.

Midwifery history does not provide a clear description of the connections between midwives and witchcraft (Oakley and Houd 1990). While there is no proof that midwives were also witches, many women were sacrificed to the ideals of the church and the state, which combined forces to eradicate the 'evil' of the time. However, it has been deduced that the terms 'woman', 'witch', 'midwife' and 'wisewoman' were used interchangeably, and that these people all fell within the category of 'a great multitude of ignorant persons' (1990: 25–26).

The witch hunts and the rise of medicine are considered to be the two main reasons why midwives' practice became more and more regulated. From a beginning of autonomous practice in the care of mothers and babies, midwives became subordinated to the medical model as 'obstetric nurses'. It is interesting, however, that the first men involved in the care of labouring women were barber surgeons who were called in by the midwives to perform destructive surgery on obstructed dead fetuses. It was not until the seventeenth century, when forceps were developed, that barber surgeons were present to assist in live births (Kitzinger 1991). As women were excluded from education, the barber surgeons and the physicians were men, and thus the male domination of midwifery was set into train.

The relationship between nursing and midwifery has also been affected by male-dominated medicine. The controlling influence of nurses by doctors was established by the time of Florence Nightingale, and the biomedical view of illness became entrenched, favouring the reduction of people to their smallest and most manageable parts. In the last 30 years or so of the twentieth century, midwifery has struggled to regain its power and autonomy and to disassociate itself from medicine and nursing. Midwifery has been keen to rid itself of the biomedical view of people, and the perspective that pregnancy, labour and delivery are disease states requiring active medical monitoring and intervention. Successive research and reviews of midwifery practice (Brown and Lumley 1994; Cunningham 1993; Rothwell 1996; Sullivan and Weitz 1998; World Health

Organisation 1985) have emphasised women's dissatisfaction with maternity services and have called for women-centred birth processes (Couves 1995).

Which of the previous definitions of midwifery best suit your definition?
How and why do they suit your definition?

Midwives

Midwives work with mothers and their partners and families throughout the various phases of the pregnancy, birth and postnatal periods. With their knowledge and skills, midwives facilitate the processes surrounding birth for the general well-being of all the people concerned. Experienced midwives work in seemingly effortless ways to bring together all components of the pregnancy, birth and postnatal periods into a process which is perceived as a continuous human event by women, their partners, family and friends. The work of midwifery has great value in creating those conditions in which mothers and others feel 'cared for' by midwives. Midwives are key people for women facing birth and child care afterwards and, sometimes, for those facing lost hopes and dreams. Midwifery practice is to be valued for its ability to make a difference in the lives of these women and the people to whom they relate.

Midwives are busy ensuring that all of the work is done safely and thoroughly. Much of their work life involves repetition, because each new mother has her own particular concerns and midwives need to accommodate these concerns, whilst ensuring that the standard care practices are followed in relation to the needs of the mother, baby and family unit. With so much to do and with so much need for repetition, midwives may develop a robot-like approach to much of their work. Developing habitual practices to deal with the sheer load and familiarity of everyday work can be useful in managing on a practical level, but it can also be detrimental in that midwifery becomes taken for granted: everyday tasks are not examined critically to find issues seated in them and ways in which they might be changed.

ORGANISATIONS AS WORK SETTINGS

Organisations are business or administrative collectives united through the pursuit of goals, such as profits and outputs. If they are not in private practice, nurses and midwives may be employed by health care organisations. The complexity of nursing and midwifery practice is intensified by the nature and effects of the organisations in which clinicians work, because the history and culture of these collectives present sets of rights and privileges, as well as constraints and challenges. Organisations are so influential in industrialised societies, and they have so much potential for interest, that they are described in organisational theory. A student of organisational theory may access this information through business, management and other professional courses, tracing themes that describe human behaviour in organisations, such as needs, drives, motivation, leadership, personality behaviour, work groups and the management of change (Anderson 1996).

Proponents of organisational theory claim that organisations have changed over time. Organisational structures and processes have moved 'from the centralised control of bureaucracies' in the 1950s and 1960s 'to shared decision-making through consultation and participative management' in the 1970s and 1980s, to the 1990s focus on 'best practice, customer-focused action and outcomes; and the manager's role as a researcher, teacher and enabler of creativity' (Anderson 1996: 30).

Max Weber (in Hoy and Miskel 1982), an influential sociologist, undertook foundational work in describing bureaucracies in the 1950s. He said that bureaucracies offered the benefits of division of labour and efficiency through specialisation, as rewards to workers for their compliance to the organisation. For example, the bureaucracy expected employees to comply with the authority of hierarchy, took objective decisions based on facts, demonstrated co-ordination and continuity through rules and regulations, and offered job protection through well-defined organisational career pathways. In effect, bureaucratic organisation offered benefits to workers at the expense of their autonomy and creativity.

Shared decision-making denoted a focus on the human relations movement, which shifted from autocratic to democratic organisational structures and processes. Communication and negotiation were the 'flavour' of the day and the intention was to increase employee job satisfaction through a sense of belonging and contributing to the organisation.

The present trend towards best practice, customer-focused action and outcomes, and the expanded role of managers, incorporates communication and accountability. Interestingly, the present organisational trends espouse shared decision-making with customers, but when you look closely, power resides ultimately within the authority of the organisational hierarchy. Some nurses and midwives might argue that their workplace is a hybrid of the three forms of organisation, or some even may even claim that their work organisation most closely resembles a bureaucracy.

Regardless of the work settings in which nurses and midwives are employed, the organisation will have a direct bearing on their potential to practise in the ways they might choose ideally. For example, Steve Kermode (1994) cautions that the organisation is a problem for the professionalisation of nursing. He warns that 'perhaps the key issue emerging from any examination of the work of professions in organisations is the conflict between autonomy and accountability' (1994: 114). On the basis of arguments that nursing is struggling to achieve professional status and organisations are expecting more and more accountability through specialisation, quantification and computers, he warns that the achievement of professional autonomy may be obstructed by health care organisations. Interestingly, in Kermode's estimation, organisations such as hospitals have not shifted from bureaucratic structures and processes. In fact, his final statements relating to the 'increasing bureaucratisation of work' warn (1994: 116) that:

> bureaucratisation has the very real possibility of diminishing the quality of the working lives of a broad range of professional occupations. For those seeking to maintain their work activities at a functional level which is above that of highly regulated process work, there is need to confront the role of the organisation in managing and controlling their work processes. This is an imperative which cannot be ignored by nurses (and midwives).

How effective are the communication patterns in your workplace?

In your opinion, to what extent does power reside with the people with authority in your organisational hierarchy?

Do you agree with Steve Kermode that organisations such as hospitals have not shifted from bureaucratic structures and processes? Write an argument supporting or refuting his position.

THE NATURE OF WORK CONSTRAINTS

Work is a complex situation in which there are many variables, such as people with different motives, ways of working and ways of interacting, and different events with many possible outcomes. With so much at stake, it is no wonder that 'things go wrong' in nursing and midwifery. You may find it relatively easy to blame yourself when work 'goes wrong', if you do not take time to reflect on the nature and effects of all the variables operating in given situations in which you are involved. When you ask: 'Why are things the way they are?' you will begin to see that there are many constraints in work settings that weigh against you giving the kind of care you might ideally choose to give. A critical appraisal may show you that your work practices can be different when constraints are acknowledged and worked on intentionally and systematically.

The world in which you exist and act as a nurse or midwife cannot help but be influenced by cultural, economic, historical, personal, political and social constraints, which may affect the ways in which you are able to interpret and act at any given moment. The realisation that you are not the only 'thing that can go wrong' in your practice may free you from bitter self-recriminations and raise your awareness to be able to transform some or all of those conditions.

Cultural constraints refer to the determinants that hold people in patterns of interaction within groups based on their shared symbols, rituals and practices. Economic constraints refer to a lack of money and the resources money can provide.

Historical constraints are those factors that have been inherited in a setting which remain unquestioned because of the precedence of time and convention. Personal constraints have to do with unique features about people, shaped by influences in their lives, into which they may or may not have insights. Political constraints are about the power, competition and contention in home and work relationships in day-to-day life. The habitual features of the setting and the ways in which people define themselves in those settings may constitute social constraints. People's daily lives can have some or all of these constraints, depending on the features of the time, place and people in them.

Do you have any cultural, economic, historical, personal, political and social constraints in your practice?
What are they?
Write down as many examples as you can. Talk with other nurses and midwives to explain the nature of the work constraints. Ask them what they think. Add to your list any other constraints they can identify. Keep your list, because this handbook shows you how to deal with constraints through reflective practice.

Looking at your own practice in order to raise your awareness about your own values and action encourages you to shift your focus outwards towards the context in which you work and how you interact there. When you ask the question: 'What or whose interests are being served?' you shift the focus away from yourself to reflect on cultural, economic, historical, political and social constraints issues that may be affecting your practice. This book will help you to work through this process.

ISSUES NURSES AND MIDWIVES OFTEN FACE

The challenges of work create issues that nurses and midwives may choose to face or ignore. Reflective processes will assist you to identify your practice issues and to work through them.

You may be wondering about the kinds of issues to which I'm referring, so the following section will give you an idea of the possibilities which can occur for nurses and midwives. Some of these issues are interrelated and may have been mentioned previously. It is important to realise that I am not suggesting these issues will necessarily be apparent in everyone's practice, but some of them may resonate with you as being important to you as you learn to become a reflective practitioner.

Daily habits and routines

Work can be satisfying and meaningful or it can be repetitive and tedious, wherever it happens. For example, at home, the daily round of making beds, washing dishes and preparing meals can become so commonplace that it stifles imagination and leads to a checklist approach of 'do this, and this, then that, and then it is over'. In paid work such as nursing and midwifery, a similar phenomenon can happen in response to repetitive tasks. Work can become entrenched in routines and habits such as 'make the beds, do the sponges, showers and baths, check on fluid and food intake', and so on. Daily habits and routines serve their purposes because they get the essential work done, but they can also become a source of practical and emotional numbness, in that the doing of the tasks becomes paramount and the people receiving the care become secondary considerations. When work is a checklist, routine and boring, or a source of constant anxiety, people become viewed as procedures and are easy to dismiss thoughtlessly, with little appreciation for how or why the tasks are being done. Daily habits and routines are a rich area for reflection, because they show you why you are practising in taken-for-granted ways and how you might be able to make some changes, given the constraints under which you work.

Do you have daily work habits and routines that you don't question?

What are they?

What do you assume should not or cannot be changed?

Write some thoughts in your journal so that you will refer back to them later.

Ideal versus real practice

Ideally, life and work would be nirvana, but in reality this is not always—or ever—so. Yearning for ideal conditions is a fairly common human tendency, and it is understandable given that we are living in an imperfect world. Wanting aspects of life and work to be ideal has interesting roots in what we have learned from childhood and adult experiences from agencies of socialisation such as the family, schools, religious affiliations and other social and cultural influences. For example, if you think that, ideally, 'all people are good', you may be challenged when you are involved in nursing and midwifery interactions with people such as patients, families and other health care workers who have motives that do not fit your definition of 'good'. Even in the face of blatant contradictions of your ideals you may try to hang on to them, to preserve some sense of personal integrity. When personal ideals are shattered in practice you may experience all kinds of emotions, such as loss, anger, confusion, helplessness, loss of self-esteem, loss of sense of purpose, and so on.

Do you have ideals which you try to hold in your work?
    What happens to you when your ideals are challenged by work constraints?
    Write some sentences about how you feel and why.

Reflective practice can assist you to see what parts of your work are based on ideals, and whether they are realisable in the face of work constraints. You may discover that daily practice falls short of your ideals, thus establishing what can become 'relatively ideal' for you, and how you may be able to achieve these ideals in your given situation.

Self-blaming

When things go wrong and you are at the centre of it, by making direct and simple connections between causes and effects, you may decide that it is your fault and resort to self-blaming, guilt and self-recrimination. Self-blaming may be based on many aspects of who you are as a person and practitioner, and the extent to which you tend to carry the blame for events in your life. While there may be occasions in which circumstances show that you have acted inappropriately, there may also be occasions on which you have been too ready to blame yourself, by not being mindful of all the other variables that were operating in the situation. Reflective processes can alert you to ponder determinants of situations and give you the means of working through them systematically so they can be managed now and prevented in the future.

Wanting to be all things to all people

Versatility is needed in nursing and midwifery practice to deal with whatever comes up in the course of daily work. However, versatility can be mistaken for invincibility and sometimes nurses and midwives may have trouble differentiating between them. If you have a need to 'be all things to all people', you may need to look at the issue of your ideal need for invincibility. Reflective processes encourage you to examine the reasons behind your need to 'be all things to all people' by asking how the situation came about, the purposes it serves and why you continue to need to be invincible in your practice.

Wanting to be perfect

One of the most important messages of years of education for practice is the need to be competent and safe. Mistakes in nursing and midwifery practice can be costly, especially if they are related to certain risky aspects of care, such as the administration of drugs or the management of life support systems. Safe practice involves up-to-date knowledge and checks and measures for ensuring that mistakes are prevented, and it is part of responsible practice to pay due attention to these strategies. For fear of making mistakes, however, some nurses and midwives may develop ritualistic modes of behaviour in which they act from a base of chronic anxiety to prevent mistakes from happening. Issues such as power, control and blaming other people may be manifestations of wanting to be perfect in all respects at work. It makes for interesting reflection to work honestly and carefully through all the possible issues that arise because of wanting to be perfect.

Can you identify instances in your work in which you tended to blame yourself, or you tried to be invincible or perfect?

Choose one of these issues and share it as a story with a work friend. She or he may like to reciprocate and share a story of her or his own. Discuss why you have tended to blame yourself, or why you tried to be invincible or perfect. Focus your discussion on any personal or professional determinants which may have influenced you to act in this way.

Struggling to be assertive

Assertive communication skills involve speaking out clearly to put a perspective plainly on view, while at the same time attending patiently and carefully to the views and needs of others. Nurses and midwives need to be assertive in their communication, in order to be effective as practitioners and to represent themselves, and the interests of their patients and their discipline, in the multidisciplinary health team. Assertive skills take practice to develop effectively and they may be mistaken for aggressive modes of communication, which come from selfish motives and have little or no regard for the feelings and beliefs of other people. If you are struggling to be assertive, you may be experiencing the effects of not finding your voice at work, leading to feelings of powerlessness and frustration. The remedy may not be as simple as assertiveness training. Quite apart from learning assertiveness skills, you may need also to discover that your lack of assertion is due to being silenced at work by powerful constraints. Reflective processes assist you to identify silencing factors and begin to take steps to lessen and eventually be freed from them.

Struggling to be an advocate

Advocacy means speaking up on someone else's behalf. Whereas you may have little trouble in being assertive about certain areas of your practice, when it comes to advocacy you may be experiencing some difficulties. Nurses and midwives need to speak up on behalf of people in their care, especially when power relationships are at play—for example, in patient–medical practitioner interactions. Hospital and clinic work situations may provide scant opportunities for patients to feel they can speak up for themselves, especially if other people with higher status seem to be too busy, unapproachable, too difficult to understand, or unwilling to communicate at the level and rate of the patient's needs. Reflective processes help you understand why advocacy is difficult for you in relation to the constraints under which you are working. You may find that being an advocate has deeper foundations than you first imagined and is not as simple as not being able to speak up on someone else's behalf because of shyness or other forms of reluctance.

Think about the word 'struggle'. What does it mean to you? Look up a dictionary to see how its definition fits with how you interpret the word.

If and when you struggle to be assertive at work, how does it feel?

If and when you struggle to be an advocate at work, how does it feel?

What constrains you from being more assertive or from acting as an advocate?

Write or tell a story a story about not being assertive at work.

Now write or tell the same story, but this time imagine yourself being assertive.

What changed in the second story?

The nurse/midwife–doctor game

There is a recognised phenomenon in nursing and midwifery practice called the nurse/midwife–doctor game (Stein 1967), in which nurses or midwives play a game of not wishing to tell doctors what to do, at the same time giving them subtle hints devoid of patronising tone and intentions, to direct them towards appropriate diagnosis or management of the patient.

Does this game ring a bell with you? Have you ever 'danced' around direct statements about diagnosis and treatment because you realise that this is not your responsibility? More importantly, have you ever reflected on why you play the game and perpetuate its traditions? Write some responses to these questions.

The nurse/midwife–doctor game is an issue for rich reflection, as it informs you about the pressures under which you work that cause you to conform to set expectations and rituals in relation to doctors. You may also get to the point where you ask yourself why you continue to promote the status quo and if, how, when and why interactions could be managed differently. This book guides you in reflecting on this and related issues.

Collegial relations

Relations between nurses and nurses, and midwives and midwives can have very little joy initially or ever, or reasonably happy relations can sour and deteriorate due to all kinds of unexamined issues, such as lack of acknowledgement, jealousy, lack of sharing of knowledge and expertise, and the old-time 'evergreen' horizontal violence. Many of the issues are self-evident. You may identify readily with feeling that your good work is unnoticed, that jealousy is an unexpressed but possible motive for poor collegial relations, and that people with knowledge and expertise may be unwilling to share it for reasons of their own, often connected to their need for recognition and power. Horizontal violence (Duffy 1995; Glass 1997) means a lashing outwards and laterally against one's own group and it is often associated with the need to overpower and subordinate others. As you can see, this mixed bag of issues about collegial relations is full of strong and influential motives, emotions and behaviours. A systematic critique of the factors that cause nurses and midwives to behave in negative ways against each other may help to unravel the threads that have bound clinicians in professional animosity and provide a means whereby some of these issues can be addressed and amended.

Have you ever lashed out against another nurse or midwife?
Has another nurse or midwife ever lashed out against you?
Why do you think horizontal violence happens in caring professions?

Organisational and health care system problems

Organisational problems and changes in the health care system, such as short staffing, bed and ward closures, communication breakdowns, lack of acknowledgement and support from administration, downsizing and rationalisation of services, and the introduction of new monitoring and management systems such as case mix, diagnosis-related groups, quality assurance and competency standards are just a few examples of the many and varied changes in health care organisations as reflected by shifts in the health care system at large.

Not far beneath the surface you will most often find political and economic motives driving the changes. As a nurse or midwife, you may find that these problems impact on you and your work life directly in the form of increased workloads, and higher expectations that you will scale the career ladder and extend your qualifications and administrative and research output. You may also be noticing that, while you are trying to adjust to these pressures, you are receiving minimal support from the people around you, who are also scrambling to keep their jobs and fulfil the sets of expectations that have been imposed on them. All of this does not make for cordial work relations, and communication across the organisation can become distorted and exceedingly difficult to maintain at an effective level. This hot-bed of discontent is the very place in which reflective processes shine, as they provide a systematic approach for making sense of how things came to be and how they could be different.

Professional identity problems

Professional identity problems are related to all kinds of other issues that arise as part of work life and they mainly amount to nurses and midwives feeling unworthy as people and practitioners. Your feelings of unworthiness may spring from many causes and you will be the only person who can say what these are. Possibilities for feeling this way may be that, at any one time, you do not know everything, you cannot be everywhere, you cannot fix everything, and you are not loved by everyone. These very large self-expectations weigh heavily on any person, and in a work setting they are the foundation of burnout, 'nervous breakdown' (or 'nervous breakthrough', as a friend of mine says), and threats—or follow through in—leaving the profession. As this problem is so large and lies at the basis of a happy personal and work life, you will notice that it is the first hurdle on the road to becoming a reflective practitioner. You will find that the first reflective task is to think about yourself and your rules for life, to sort out what you have idealised and applied to your work life. Although this first step may not solve all your feelings of unworthiness, it will alert you to their presence and assist you in getting started on the process of building a positive sense of personal and professional worth.

The issues raised in this section are some of many which may be faced by nurses and midwives.

What other issues do you face in your practice?

What strategies are you using to overcome these issues?

How successful have your strategies been?

SOME STORIES EXEMPLIFYING ISSUES

In this chapter I have described the nature and effects of nursing and midwifery and some of the issues that arise for nurses and midwives in the course of their work. You were also introduced to three clinicians who have used the reflective processes in this book. To exemplify the kinds of issues that may become sources of reflection for you, I now offer three stories. Carol, Michael and Esther will each describe an incident at work and I highlight the practice issues they faced. Please note that I have not changed anything in their transcripts, other than the areas they requested of me, so you will find each person's own unedited writing style, practice-specific language and abbreviations in these stories.

Carol's story about newborn death

Listened to report, allocated half of ward. Two staff present. Checked all of patients.

One patient, Mrs G (having Cervagen termination for fetal abnormalities). Eighteen weeks' gestation. 10pm evening sister performed VE, bulging forewaters, Cervagen not inserted, it could be soon.

After checking all my patients I sat with Mr and Mrs G for a while ascertaining contractions and their disposition. Continued four to five minutes, nil present in anus. Husband in attendance.

2300—Feeling slightly more pressure. I discussed with the couple what to expect delivery wise and then what the baby might look like and they told me about the ultrasound and what they were expecting themselves.

Patient moved on to floor on her knees as the back ache getting a bit much.

I mentioned they had had a hard time in the unit this day as a full-term baby had died in second stage. This opened up conversation more and we talked about people's reactions and mother said 'You can always have another one' and the inappropriateness of this statement and perhaps grandparents in particular may have a lot of difficulty with this situation.

2320—Baby born still inside the sac and pla-

centa dropped out on top all intact. The parents were quite fascinated as the membranes were very tough and difficult to break. The three of us looked at the baby and the husband cried. Baby's eyes were wide open, not usual for this gestation.

Over the next few hours I checked the woman and then took photos and footprints, handprints of baby. Dressed it in a cute nightie I found. Baby a bit smelly after a while and into the fridge.

Another comment by the mother a few hours afterward. 'Did he have any eyelids? He doesn't look peaceful.'

Reflections

Oh no not another one and hoping it would be born on another shift or at least in labour ward, but no I am stuck with yet another dead malformed one. But I had done numerous before, it was just a job which had to be done.

My leading questions and explanations allowed the parents to talk and discuss their fears, feelings and express emotions.

The woman was very calm as she said she had had a bit of time to grieve. Husband cried when he saw him. I don't think I had any emotion, just flat and the ward work needed to be done.

When delivering and looking at baby with parents I try to be quiet, respectful and allow them enough time to talk with each other as well as supporting them.

I was taken aback with the question re the baby's eyes being open and him not being peaceful. In my mind he was the picture of an alien and for myself will I be able to sleep tomorrow without waking up with aliens before my face? The next night I was angry at the pathetic inconsistent follow-up *offered to maternity staff. Last evening they had had the incident of the fresh stillbirth and they had arranged a debriefing for all staff involved. I had delivered a dead baby as well. Treatment is pathetic anyway. I know I have to get my own support. My family are supportive and I also went out to lunch with the female registrar. We talked a little about the debriefing as she was the doctor involved with the fresh stillbirth. She refused to go to the debriefing. I was able to express to her the fact I had delivered a dead baby as well and we agreed the lack of follow-up there. Nurses, and especially midwives, have to cope with death, often unfair congenital abnormalities, there is no reason, there is no cure. Medicine is incapable of fixing these things. Medicine has no answers.*

Practice issues in Carol's story

In this story Carol related the incident of a newborn death in utero due to fetal abnormalities. When I looked at her account I noticed some statements which gave me clues about the kinds of issues she faced in this story.

Carol commented on the unenviable work she had to face, when she was involved in yet another birth of a dead baby. Although she did not enjoy the work, she was accustomed to it and knew it needed to be done. She also reflected on her emotion, or lack of it, and the busyness of her job.

Carol was angry about the lack of support for staff after a delivery of a dead baby. She also noted that nurses and midwives are expected to cope, no matter what happens.

In summary, the issues raised by this story include the unenviable nature of midwives' work and the necessity for it to be done. Emotional issues were secondary to the busyness of the job. Lack of support for staff after a delivery of a dead baby, and the necessity to always cope, were also issues which could be acknowledged and clarified through reflective processes.

Are there any issues in this story which resonate with your own?
    What are they?
    How have you dealt with them in your work?

Michael's story about management versus clinical

Having recently returned to the bedside after six years in management, all the managers and go-getters around the hospital think I am mad. For me it has been a truly enlightening and stress-free experience. Combined with the journalling and reflecting on my practice I now remember how much I used to enjoy clinical practice.

My management experience has been in the cut-throat private hospital sector where budgets are constantly being cut, targets being raised and the expectation is that the quality of care remains high. Quality is a grossly overused term in the private hospital sector, I feel, and is something that I have seen often compromised for the sake of the dollar.

As a Unit Manager for five years working within the restraints of a budget I feel I was in a no-win situation constantly. I was answerable to management if staffing lists were high. Answerable to staff if staffing levels were too low, but rarely had to answer to the patients, who despite what level of care they received, remained largely non-complaining.

My most effective means of managing I have found in this time is to lead by example as keeping my staff happy is everything to me. If nursing staff aren't happy, everybody suffers. I always maintain I will not ask any nurse to do anything I would not do myself.

At present I am working alongside clinicians who have been subjected to staffing cuts that I have been part of implementing. Whilst they have all been nice to me and most realised that I was not responsible for staff cuts, I know that there have been a few people waiting for me to complain about lack of staff or not being able to do things well.

Thankfully I have been able to work within the levels set without any problem. I work really hard and go home exhausted, but generally happy about what I have been able to achieve.

I have for five years not received any significant positive feedback—sure management pat you on the back if you are saving dollars. But staff rarely take the time to say to their Unit Manager— job well done. In my last role everybody waited until my resignation was in before they began to let me know how they had appreciated what I had tried to do for them. Up until my resignation all I heard was about their frustration with not being able to achieve what they wanted to. (The hospital was going through a sale and money was very tight— Heads of Department were asked from time to time not to bank their pay cheques to give you an indication of how tight money was.) My role was to keep nursing staff happy and productive, something which was achieved well but unfortunately I didn't get to realise how well until after I had left.

At this point in time I am working part-time night duty. I like the nights because of the level of basic nursing care you can achieve and the relationships you develop with the patients. I get immense satisfaction out of seeing results for the work— patients walking, getting better and going home.

Most of all I get a kick out of the feedback direct from patients.

Tonight at the start of the shift a patient who came in for a vaginal repair and ended up with a PE left a message for me to see her before she settled for the night. Her nights have been very unsettled due to pain from the PE and worrying about all the information being fed to her from different levels. She has been on warfarin and given the pathology anticoagulant info book. This book covers every possible scenario so as not to land its publishers in a law court, however by the time the average layperson has read the book they find it hard to believe they can be on warfarin and lead a normal life. Many nights were spent explaining the warfarin therapy over sips of warm Milo and demystifying the information being received.

I went to visit Enid as requested as she is being discharged tomorrow. In the middle of a general discussion I had told Enid I was going to Washington DC this week. When I got there Enid had bought (or had her husband buy for me) a copy of the Lonely Planet guide to Washington DC so that I could read about the places she had suggested I visit whilst in Washington.

If this is acceptance, being part of the healing process, being visible or being acknowledged—I'm there!

These situations mean more to me than any management/administrative achievements. This is what I wanted for myself back in my first year of training watching my father die. Making a difference to somebody's stay, helping them work their way through the fog that is our health system and come out the other end feeling better for the nursing contact along the way.

Identify the issues in this story, with which Michael grappled in his practice as an administrator and clinician. Have you ever had similar issues? If so, how did you deal with these issues?

Practice issues in Michael's story

Some issues I identified relate to economic constraints, lack of support and lack of acknowledgment. Michael wrote of economic constraints on giving nursing care and the dilemma that placed him in as a Unit Manager. He also noted his problem in working in clinical practice and the blame he felt was directed towards him. Lack of positive feedback was another issue identified in Michael's story.

Issues relating to economic constraints, lack of support and lack of acknowledgment can be dealt with by effectively using reflective processes. This does not mean that they disappear as issues, but rather that they become more manageable in the light of new insights which surface through systematic reflection.

Esther's story about inadequate epidural anaesthesia

I was caring for a woman in labour with her first baby. The babe was in the posterior position and progress was agonisingly slow for the woman. I used every trick in the book to aid her comfort and empower her to diminish the increasing back pain experienced during contractions. However, finally, she couldn't take anymore. We were in one of the two birthing rooms in hospital and it was early evening. The room was peaceful and smelt good from the aromatherapy massage blend I'd been using on the woman's back and belly, either massaging myself or getting her husband to do it.

So, eventually the woman requested an epidural

anaesthetic to get rid of the pain. My heart sank! Ideologically, I would turn myself inside out to help labouring women to do without epidurals. However, as long as they are making an informed choice, I am happy to support their decisions. There is one major flaw here though, and that is the medical practitioner who actually inserts the epidural catheter and commences the anaesthesia. This general practitioner has GP anaesthetic rights to the hospital, despite the fact that he no longer provides any regular anaesthetic service on a regular basis. He continues to be reaccredited for anaesthetics and obstetrics (despite only reaching about one-third of the number of deliveries required per triennium for reaccreditation for the Health Service). He is totally inept in both specialties, and seemingly has no compassion, empathy or ethical belief structures, in that he continues to provide care which, to say the least, is not in the best interests of either woman or baby!! As this GP is the senior partner of the medical practice where two junior partners work who acquire probably the majority of obstetric clients in the town, and who, by the way, offer a particularly interventionist, old-fashioned, medically dominated type of obstetric care (that's another story!!), he is invariably called in to 'do' the epidurals!

And so, to continue the story. He attempted to insert an epidural catheter. I was on the other side, facing the woman, supporting her, checking maternal and fetal obs, regulating the IVI, etc. Another midwife, who I'd called in to help, was assisting the GP. The catheter was inserted—I looked over and noted blood in the catheter. The GP took the catheter out, poked around the woman's spine, muttering to himself (his usual form of communication) and then commenced to reinsert the same catheter, despite being offered a new catheter by the midwife assisting. We both raised our eyebrows and looked to the younger GP to see what he would do. Nothing happened! The catheter was reinserted and protocols for the anaesthesia commenced. After about 15–20 minutes, the woman was experiencing virtually no relief, was using nitrous oxide intermittently, and the GP/obs decided on transfer to our Base Hospital for 'failure to progress'. Before transfer, the epidural was 'topped up', still with minimal effectiveness. I accompanied the woman in the ambulance, and she used nitrous oxide the whole way—a 40-minute trip. She kept asking me the reason the epidural wasn't working. I suggested she asked the GP!

I left her in the capable hands of the midwives and returned to [home]. As is my usual practice, I rang the Base in a couple of hours to find out what was happening, if the woman had delivered, etc. At that stage, she was still in labour, was being augmented and monitored, and the epidural catheter had been removed and reinserted. Epidural anaesthesia was now effective! She finally delivered vaginally!

The next afternoon, the GP/obs who had admitted the woman was at the desk. I asked whether he'd heard about the outcome of the labour/transfer, and when he said no, I told him. There were several people at the desk, at least two other midwives. I commented that the epidural had been ineffective all the way to the Base Hospital and he rejected that statement, saying that it had 'seemed' to be working a bit before transfer, this despite the fact that the woman was writhing around on the ambulance trolley when out of reach of the nitrous oxide!

I then suggested that the GP who had inserted the epidural might think about ceasing this service (for want of a better word!)—disservice would be better, as he did them so infrequently that they rarely were effective. I also noted the blood in the epidural catheter and the fact that the catheter was reused!

A deathly hush enveloped the desk area. No one moved or uttered a word, despite the fact that several staff, including the midwives had been commenting on the unprofessional, inept practice of this GP prior to his partner arriving on the scene! The GP became very defensive and angry and one of the other midwives suggested that it was inappropriate to discuss the incident any further at the desk. I decided not to pursue the incident further at that time, and left the desk area, where nursing staff were smoothing the ruffled feathers of the GP.

I was furious regarding the lack of peer support, and said as much later. Blank faces, blushes and turned backs greeted me. I resolved to see my hospital manager regarding the issue of inappropriate/ineffective practice of the GPs (again!!). Again, the manager agreed, again nothing happened, despite representations to the medical reaccreditation committee and the Health Service obstetricians and anaesthetists (via the Health Service pain management/epidural expert, clinical nurse specialist). For some reasons, lack of medical expertise wins over optimal care!!

In the meantime, the GP/obs refused to talk to me, and any communication was effected through a third person for some time. About a week after this incident, the GP/anaesthetist in question enquired regarding the condition of one of his patients, for whom I was caring. I provided some information, including care suggestions from the physiotherapist. He said 'I don't give a stuff what the physio says and I don't give a stuff what you say'. I said

'There's no need to be rude . . .' He replied, *'Well, you're rude to the doctors.'* I realised very quickly that his partner must have told him what had transpired the previous week regarding my comments about his practice. I commented that I was not being rude and had the right to my own professional opinion and that I was not going to continue the conversation any longer. I walked into our staff room shaking and then bawled my eyes out, as much from frustration and the injustice of it all, as anything! Another RN asked what was wrong, and on hearing the story, supported me and suggested I see the hospital manager again. I did, he was supportive and interceded on my behalf, which meant that relations between myself and the two GPs are now superficially cordial. However, nothing has changed regarding the practice issues!!

Practice issues in Esther's story

Esther's story is about finding voice in midwife–doctor relationships, but it also includes issues about working with other midwives. The major issue related to the perception of doctor incompetence and what to do about it. The 'raised eyebrows' she describes were the shared message between midwives that the reinsertion of the same catheter was inappropriate. It is interesting to reflect on why the midwives chose non-verbal communication in preference to open statements of dismay at the inappropriateness of management.

When she spoke up, Esther was drawn into open confrontation with the doctor and received no support from her colleagues. Esther also explained the retaliative outcome of speaking up.

In summary, Esther's issues were located in midwife–doctor relationships, but they also included issues about working with other midwives. Doctor incompetence and what to do about it was the main issue; however, struggling to be assertive was also apparent in the 'raised eyebrows' non-verbal exchange between the midwives. Another issue was the need to witness unnecessary pain as a result of inappropriate management and to be honour bound not to impugn the doctor. On speaking up, Esther faced the issue of open confrontation with the doctor, no support from her colleagues, and retaliative consequences from doctors. All of these issues can be explored in depth using reflective processes, which will be explained in detail later in this book.

Can you identify any other issues in this story?
What does this story suggest to you about the nature of midwifery practice?

SUMMARY

In this chapter I introduced two midwives and one nurse, all of whom are engaged in practice on a regular basis. I described the nature of nursing and midwifery according to some definitions in the literature and suggested that working in organisations increases the complexity of work. I noted that, although the trend in the 1990s has been towards best practice, customer-focused action and outcomes, and the expanded role of managers, hospitals may still resemble bureaucracies. I suggested that your work world cannot help but be influenced by cultural, economic, historical, political and social constraints, which may affect the ways in which you are able to interpret and act in any given moment. Work issues were explored, such as daily habits and routines, ideal versus real practice, self-blaming, wanting to be all things to all people, wanting to be perfect, struggling to be assertive, struggling to be an advocate, the nurse/midwife–doctor game, collegial relations, organisational and health care system problems, and professional identity problems. Finally, Carol, Michael and Esther exemplified some work issues through their stories. My main intention for this chapter was to show how and why nursing and midwifery are complex occupations requiring careful attention to many aspects through reflective practice.

3

Getting ready to reflect

In this chapter I describe the basic essentials you need to prepare for reflection. To get you ready for your journey into reflective territories, I give you some more information about reflective practice, and supply you with a kitbag of strategies to help you on your way. I suggest that you need determination, courage and a sense of humour, and a critical friend who will help you on your journey by drawing your attention to points of interest along the way so that you can appreciate them more.

KNOWLEDGE OF REFLECTIVE PRACTICE

The major theoretical ideas on which reflective practice is based are introduced in this book. Even so, for your convenience, some of the literature will be reiterated here, so that you can get a grasp on what matters most when you are thinking about becoming a reflective practitioner. Probably the most notable name in the reflective practice literature is Donald Schön, who was a champion of practitioners in his unswerving belief that they were capable of reflective thought which could lead to changes in practice.

Schön emphasised the idea that reflection is a way in which professionals can bridge the theory–practice gap, based on the potential of reflection to uncover knowledge in and on action (Schön 1983). He had an unswerving belief in the working intelligence of practitioners, and their potential to make sense of their work in a theoretical way, even though they might tend to play down their knowledge. He referred to tacit knowledge, or knowing-in-action, as the kind of knowledge practitioners have, of which they may not be entirely aware. He wrote:

> Often we cannot say what it is that we know. When we try to describe it we find ourselves at a loss, or we produce descriptions that are obviously inappropriate. Our knowing is ordinarily tacit, implicit in our patterns of action and in the feel for the stuff with which we are dealing. It seems right to say that our knowing is in our action.

The practical outcome of what Schön had to say about reflective practice is that it can enable nurses and midwives to articulate what it is they know and how they have come to know it. When nurses and midwives make explicit their knowing-in-action, they can inevitably use this awareness to enliven and change their practice. Whatever the outcomes, reflection has, at the very least, the potential to be transformative to some degree; therefore, it could be considered a worthwhile activity. Donald Schön also argued that reflection is not a simple process and that practitioners need coaching and reflective diaries as tools for dealing with practice problems (Schön 1987).

Do you agree with Donald Schön that, as a practitioner, you cannot always say what you know? If your answer is 'Yes!' you may have a sense that your actions are guided by knowledge you may be unable to express. Take heart! This book intends to help you make more explicit to you some of those hidden aspects of your practice.

In the meantime, think of any occasions at work after which you were impressed with your practice and thought to yourself something like: 'Wow! That went well! How did I do that? How did I know that?'

Find a place where you can talk out aloud and speak freely in response to these trigger questions:

- What went well?
- Why did it go well?
- Where did it happen?
- Who was involved?
- How were you involved?
- What did you do?
- Why did you do what you did?
- What were you thinking at the time?
- What do you think about it now?

Bear in mind that you may not be able to bring all of your knowledge to the surface in your responses to this reflector. However, you will become more accustomed to freer thinking, and thereby improve your ability in connecting your thoughts to reach fresh insights about your practice.

Another name which has been linked to reflective practice since its emergence in education literature is Boud (1985: 20), who suggests that reflection has the potential to recreate the totality of experience and that the 'outcomes of reflection may be a personal synthesis, integration and appropriation of knowledge, the validation of personal knowledge, a new affective state, or the decision to engage in some further action'.

Boud's quote is in compact language, but it means that reflection has the potential to affect you in a complete way, and this may be through creating a new awareness of yourself, in helping you to bring together and use knowledge, to work out for yourself what counts as truth, to take on a different emotional stance, or to make up your mind to do something else. This set of outcomes is based on a personal experience with far-reaching positive consequences for the person who engages in reflection. It is not difficult to ascertain the message 'between the lines' though: that this kind of personal metamorphosis requires some effort on the part of the person seeking these personal benefits—it will not just happen as if by magic.

According to Greenwood (1993) and Conway (1994), coaching promotes collaborative knowing. It is referred to by Belenky et al. (1986: 33) as 'connected teaching', which encourages a cooperative communication style between the instructor and participants. Establishing a climate of collaboration during the learning process prepares learners for the changes they identify as being needed in the workplace. In a similar way, in this book I hope to set up a guided approach which encourages you to keep on going. If you use this guide in collaboration with a selection of critical friends and peers, you will be able to set up a situation of connection and cooperation.

A number of strategies have been suggested in the literature for the documentation of reflection—for example, journal writing, metaphor analysis, storytelling and portfolio development (Caffarella and Barnett 1994). I suggest many ways of reflecting in this book and the more creative you can be in selecting means to suit you, the better it will be for you. Becoming a reflective practitioner takes time and effort. Newell (1992), in his critique of the use of reflection in nursing, concedes that mentors and support persons need time in training and support themselves. I imagine that you will be using this book in conjunction with a course of study, or at your own pace as you attend work. Please ensure that you access as much support and other avenues of training as you can as you develop reflective practice. I have suggested some support systems in Chapter 11 which may be helpful.

A KITBAG OF STRATEGIES

If you have heard about reflective practice before, you may have gained the impression that it is about keeping a journal or log of some sort. Even though I think writing is an important means of recording your thoughts and feelings, it is not the only way to aid your reflection. I'm hoping that this news may come as a pleasant surprise if you are someone who has trouble writing things down. In this section I suggest ways in which reflection can be stimulated and recorded for later analysis. It is important that you keep a record of your practice stories for reviewing and this is possible through writing, audiotaping, creating music, dancing, drawings, montage, painting, poetry, pottery, quilting, singing and videotaping. Any of these methods may be used alone or in combination.

Writing

Keeping a journal is a favoured means of storing experiences. To prepare for writing, you need an exercise writing book or a computer or typewriter. For any of these writing methods you also require time, effort and imagination, but let's leave these last three requisites to one side as they will be highlighted later.

Returning to the handwriting materials, I suggest that you buy a fixed-page exercise book so that you will be less likely to tear out pages when you are tempted to edit your writing. This may mean that your journal gets a bit messy, but at least it will be complete, 'warts and all'. The pen should be one which you can handle well so you can write quickly and easily.

If you are using a computer for wordprocessing, it will probably be because you can type fairly well or you have become accustomed to thinking through this kind of writing. You will most probably be aware of the usual tips for computing, such as using good quality disks and saving your document often if you do not have an automatic save function. The best hints I can give you are what to avoid.

Just type, don't edit your writing by cutting out sentences and paragraphs. Unlike wordprocessing for formal tasks such as assignments, it is a good idea to type as you think without much, if any, planning. Don't shift chunks of writing to other parts of the document to make it more grammatical or ordered. Thoughts may come in random order and themes may not be connected. This is the way some thinking happens in private, so don't try to change it or it or put it into a form to suit a wider audience.

If you are using a typewriter, it is also important for you not to try to get your writing ordered and edited so it looks nice or reads well. You need to let your typing flow with your thoughts and 'learn to live with' any disordered typing mess which may arise. You also need to keep anything you write in a self-holding folder which keeps all the pages in the order in which they were typed.

Write free flowing journal entry under the heading: 'My best day at work'. I do not want to suggest any structuring questions for this writing task, so feel free to approach it in your own way.

Audiotaping

Not everyone is blessed with a love of writing and an ability to do it easily. Fortunately, you can learn to reflect without a lot of writing. If you are really systematic in how you use other methods I'm suggesting here, you may be able to avoid writing altogether. Do you enjoy telling stories? If you do, you could tell your stories into a tape-recorder so you have a record of what you say. Once you get over the awkwardness of sitting alone and chattering away to what initially might seem like an intimidating machine, you will get into the swing of reflecting through talking. If you feel a bit silly at first, tell the tape-recorder, experience the feeling completely, and then choose to 'get over it' and value the silent gaps which may also occur. Let the words come easily and effortlessly. Also leave your words unedited by resisting the temptation to rewind and tape over certain sections.

If you are intending to use the tape recordings without any written notes to yourself, you need to develop the habit of reviewing what you said previously to make verbal remarks on successive recordings. In this way you will be able to keep a progressive record of the insights you have gained so that you can make connections to what is yet to become apparent through the reflective process. This may mean that you accumulate a lot of audiotapes, so be sure to date and label them carefully, so you know which ones to replay as the need arises. The reflective processes described in this book work just as well by audiotaping as they do by writing, as long as you review the audiotapes frequently and carefully to identify and work on connections in what you have said about your practice.

Record yourself talking about 'My worst day at work'.

Compare the written and spoken versions of your reflections and write some notes in response to these questions:

- Which form of reflection seemed easier—the written or the spoken form?
- Why was it easier?
- What are the 'pros and cons' of both methods?

Creative music

You do not have to be a musician to make music, if you let the instrument express how you are feeling and thinking. For example, you could beat out a rhythm on a drum or a drum-like substitute, shake a tambourine or a bag full of marbles, or strike randomly on a musical keyboard such as a piano, organ or xylophone. While you might make a fairly awful sound, it is important to make it. Alternatively, if you have some formal training and some musical skills, this may allow you to create a more aesthetically pleasing sound.

Why would you want to create music to help you reflect? The music may help you create sounds which represent what you are thinking, or it may allow you to let out some feelings so that you have something on which to reflect. Thoughts and feelings are components of reflection and they can become locked in if they cannot find expression. Play your music, or make your noise, and watch yourself to see what happens. You may find creative expression for feelings you are having about clinical issues and, as you are experiencing them, tune in to the thoughts you are having.

As you need a record of your reflections, write or audio- or videotape your thoughts which emerge as partial or complete stories. You might choose to tape the music you create and then use the recording machine to voice your thoughts and feelings afterwards. Alternatively, you might choose to write your reflections or use any other combinations of methods described in this section.

Once the stories start to flow through the release of music, you will have some substance on which to reflect and you can use music at any stage of the reflective process thereafter.

Dancing

If you have some means of mobility, you can dance. You do not have to be upright and bipedal to dance. People in wheelchairs and on walking aids can dance. Even if you feel like a baby elephant or paddle footed when you try to dance, give it a go anyway. The point I am making here is that you will have some difficulty making excuses for why you cannot dance. Feel it and do it. It's easy if you just let go and dance, with or without music. Move by whatever means you have and let your body show you how you feel about work issues. At the same time, as with any other creative expression, you can also notice yourself as an interested observer. The feelings and thoughts evoked by dance will be useful for reflective processes. Having been evoked, thoughts and feelings can be channelled into systematic reflective processes, which are yet to be described in this book.

Decide on ways of recording your reflections evoked or played out through dance. You could audio- or videotape the thoughts which emerge as partial or complete stories. A videotape would be especially helpful, as it could capture the dance and your reflections during or after. The recording needs to be available for reviewing, so you can make progressive reflections as new issues emerge from your practice. If dancing inspires reflection or represents what you are thinking and feeling, it may be a creative reflection possibility for you.

Drawing

You may have the ability to draw what is in your head and 'heart', but if you do not, don't worry. Think of drawing as systematic doodling and you might feel a bit more confident about using drawing as a means of reflecting. Remember also that drawings are whatever you say they represent, so they do not need to be realistic or accurate or fulfil any other artistic criterion. Whether the drawings happen spontaneously as an expression of what you are thinking and feeling, or whether they happen intentionally as a result of these processes, they can be useful in combination with interpretations which document the sense you have been able to make of your clinical experiences.

Record your responses to, or reasons for, the drawings you have made in relation to issues you are experiencing at work. Record your insights systematically in an enduring form so they can be revisited. For example, you could compile them in a book with space in between each for interpretations and insights, or you could record your reflections by speaking into a tape-recorder. If you are keeping a journal they could be incorporated into what you are writing. Do whatever feels right for you.

Draw a symbol or set of symbols to represent the person you are at home.
What have you drawn?
What is your drawing indicating about the person you are at home?
Write your responses in your journal.

Montage

A montage is a collection of images. Montages are often created from pictures, words and symbols cut out from old magazines and newspapers. If you have the time and interest in having fun with magazines, scissors and glue, making a montage might be an excellent way of assisting your reflective processes. As you search for images to express what you are thinking and feeling about clinical issues, you might find that you begin to reflect more fully, so that the montage which emerges is a comprehensive representation of the sense you are making of practice events. On the other hand, the montage may provide you with a glimpse of where further reflection may take you, and you may not make connections until later when you take previous montages out of storage to review them.

Regardless of the way in which you organise your montage-assisted reflections, you need to record your successive interpretations so that the processes described in this book can be applied to them. The connecting ideas and themes may be represented in other montages as you progress as a reflective practitioner.

Make a montage of the person you are at work.
What words, symbols and other creative representations have you used?
What is your montage indicating about the person you are at home?
Write your responses in your journal.

Painting

Watercolours, oil or acrylic paints can be used to paint a picture of your practice. It does not matter if it turns out to be a mess, because you are the painter and your painting is what you say it is. Let's face it—your painting may not be up to gallery standard, but it will be valuable for you as it can depict your responses to issues in your practice.

As you are painting, notice the colours you choose, and how you apply the paint. Tune in to what you are thinking and feeling as you paint each stroke. You can paint spontaneously in response to your emotions and thoughts or you can make deliberate strokes to structure your thinking into an image of your reflections.

Keep all your paintings and a commentary about them on tape or in a journal. Issues change over time, and you may notice that your painting style changes with them. It is important that you make sense of your paintings and incorporate those interpretations into the systematic reflective processes described in this book. Use this method for as long as it is helpful in combination with some other method which provides some written or spoken words about the meaning of the paintings and where they fit and why into your reflective practitioner experiences.

Poetry

Everyone can write poetry which has personal style and meaning. If you know any rules of poetry, by all means apply them, but even if you don't have the slightest idea of the structure of poetry, you could write some anyway.

I write poetry from time to time and I imitate the rhythm and flow of other poems I have read, or I simply put as many words along one line as I fancy. My poems may never be published, but every time I take my own poetry book off the shelf and read it, my words bring back all the thoughts and feelings I had at the time of writing. This is why I think poetry could help you as you engage in systematic reflection on your practice.

When I write poetry I let the words come as they will. Sometimes the words repeat in my head until I can find a place in which to write them. The slightest inspiration could be the basis of a poem. If you have had a hectic day at work which has stirred up a lot of emotions and thoughts, try putting them into words. Your poem might be one line or go into proportions that would make Shakespeare envious. It does not matter, just let the poem flow as long as it needs to, so that you can express the issues on your mind.

As with all creative expressions for assisting reflection, you need to record your responses to your poetry, explaining how you wrote it, why and for whom, and what it means in relation to your practice reflections. Keep all your poems and commentaries and incorporate them into the other methods you are using for reflection.

Pottery

My experience of pottery is limited, but I am not much of a painter, dancer or quilter either. I work on the idea that anything is accessible to me if I can imagine it, so here are my ideas on how I think pottery could help your reflection.

Not only is clay a wonderful medium for venting your emotions, it can form into practical or impractical shapes, forms and symbols which can represent clinical issues. If you have had a particularly terrible day at work why not experiment with clay? If you create a form spontaneously or intentionally, notice how you are feeling and the thoughts you are having in relation to work. Keep all the dried clay pieces or take a photograph and record your insights successively and weave them into future reflections.

> Why not choose one of the three Ps – painting, poetry or pottery—and follow my suggestions to reflect on this question:
> 'What issue keeps on coming up in my practice, which I feel least able to change?'
> After using one or more of the methods, record your reflections and keep them for later review.

Quilting

Quilting is a deliberate act of sewing to represent selected themes of life. The symbols are selected carefully to contribute to the whole story depicted in the quilt.

I imagine you may be thinking: 'Does Bev seriously think that I am ever going to make a quilt to represent my practice?' My answer is: 'Well, if you know how to, or you would like to learn, why not! If you become a reflective practitioner for life, you have plenty of time!'

As you sit and sew, you could reflect on each symbol, and how it relates to the whole. In between quilting you could record your reflections and 'sew' them into other methods for reflecting you may be using, such as writing or audiotaping.

Singing

By singing, I mean that you create a melody and words that come straight out of the creative space inside yourself. As with many creative tasks, this can be difficult if you are overly self-conscious. To get started, sing a song you know. This will help you get used to the sound of your own singing voice. As you will be singing in private it does not matter if you sing off key or if your lyrics are less than poetic. Just open your mouth, breathe in, and sing out spontaneously!

As this is singing with reflective practice intentions, you need some form of recording, such as audiotaping or video-taping. You can decide on your level of comfort and skill in using either of these two recording methods. Also, you need to make successive documentation of your interpretations of, and insights into, your songs and singing, noticing the words you used, the volume, pitch and mood of your singing, and your thoughts and feelings as you sang. These ideas and any more you develop along the way can be orchestrated into the other methods of reflection you are using, so that you can gain maximal effects from your reflective practice.

Videotaping

If you have ready access to video equipment, you might like to consider this as the primary medium by which to enhance your reflection. One of the obvious benefits of using this medium is that you will be able to review what and how you do. Your own non-verbal cues may be interesting for you to observe. For example, in telling some of your clinical stories, you may find that there is a substantial emotional component of which you were not fully aware. Your posture or pitch of voice may have something to tell you about yourself. When you use the reflective processes described in this book, you will discover that they require you to be as honest and frank with yourself and your work as you can. Seeing yourself respond to these questions may enhance your reflections as you ask yourself about your non-verbal and verbal self as portrayed on video.

As you need to make sense of your reflections, you need to develop a method for amassing progressive insights, questions and connections in your practice. You may choose to record these impressions directly onto the video or into some other form of semi-permanent record, such as a journal or audiotape.

A REFLECTIVE TASK

Reflection can occur through one or a combination of methods. If you have been responding to the reflectors in the book thus far, you will have been writing in your journal and talking with friends and colleagues. This is not the beginning for you as a reflective person or practitioner, as you may have already developed some of the features of reflective practice by thinking carefully about your work and life up to this point. My assumption is that, as an adult, you are reading this book with some experience of reflecting. I am also assuming that what you may require now are some processes and structures which can help you to reflect more systematically and effectively.

A process is about how to do something. In this section I suggest how you can reflect on and record your childhood memories in relation to you now as an adult and a clinician. I suggest certain processes for recording your reflection which I hope will help your thoughts flow more easily. A structure refers to the way something is organised and constructed. In this book, structure refers specifically the kinds of tasks I suggest to help you organise your thinking about your practice. The main basis of the structures are the questions I pose and the other questions you and your critical friend pose to you.

Hints for reflecting

The following suggestions are for any kind of reflection you might use in the future, such as technical, practical or emancipatory forms described in Chapters 7 to 9. These comments also relate to any methods you might use to enhance reflection, such as writing, audiotaping, videotaping or some form of creative representation such as painting, montage, drawing, quilting, pottery, poetry, singing, dancing and/or creating music.

Be spontaneous

A very important consideration to remember as you reflect is to be as spontaneous as possible in recording your thoughts and feelings. It is from the frank and honest self that important insights come. If you try to 'sanitise' these valuable parts of yourself, you will not be able to get to the 'heart' of the matter as effectively. Too many things will be left unexpressed and lack of clarity will result from gaps in the account of the experience.

Express yourself freely

As your reflections are for yourself primarily, feel free to express them as directly as you can. These are your reflections, which you may choose to share partially or wholly with a critical friend, so be as explicit as you possibly can. This might mean that you swear sometimes or admit to and represent other emotions and thoughts which express themselves in socially unacceptable or staggered, incomplete ways. It does not matter if your accounts and representations are rude at times, inaccurate in grammar or spelling, or do not conform to expected norms of your chosen language.

Remain open to ideas

Sometimes you may find some answers as you reflect, but do not jump on these insights as being absolute answers. Try to leave ideas open and treat them as tentatively as possible. Early conclusions may inhibit further insights and solutions, so be prepared for twists and turns in your thinking and for some questions that remain unanswered indefinitely.

Choose a time to suit you

You know the times of day when you feel alert and when you feel tired. Choose a time of day when you feel fresh and ready to give some quality time to thinking about your practice.

Good planning will also mean that you set time aside in your busy life for reflecting; if it is not left to chance, it may mean that you are more likely to develop regular reflective habits. In this way, you create a space in which you can reflect, where no other pressures intervene for a while.

Be prepared personally

Getting ready for reflection warrants some personal preparation. What you do will be entirely up to you, but I suggest that you feel as fresh and alert as possible, so you might like to do some favoured exercise, meditate, or experience some other form of relaxation which puts you into an attentive, imaginative mood.

Choose a reflective method

You need to keep a record of your practice stories for reviewing. Any of the methods discussed earlier, or more as you imagine them, may be used alone or in combination. All you have to do is to decide what you want to do and set it into train. If you decide that you want to adjust your reflective methods as you go, that is quite acceptable. The idea is to reflect as freely, spontaneously, deeply and comprehensively as possible, so experiment until you find the combinations of methods which suit you best.

STRUCTURES FOR REFLECTING

Reflective tasks will be structured by questions I pose in this book, or by questions posed by you or someone else. Therefore, enquiry is the basis for reflection and it is the structure on which reflection is built. This is another way of describing some of the points I make in Chapter 6, in which I introduce you to types of knowledge and reflection. All of these ideas have enquiry of some kind at their roots, because questions invoke reflection and answers promote knowledge.

This reflective task will help you to get started as a reflective practitioner and to begin the complex and lifelong business of getting to know yourself as a person and practitioner in time and context. I hope you enjoy this preparatory exercise. I invite you to use whatever method of reflecting you choose, such as writing, audiotaping or other creative ways of enhancing reflection as described in this chapter, to think about your childhood and the person and practitioner you are now.

Reflecting on your personal history

The following task gives you an opportunity to think about yourself in your own personal, social and historical context, so that you can then think about how you have come to be the person and practitioner you are now.

These questions (Smyth, 1986a) are based on those I used when I first studied reflective processes during my studies in education at Deakin University in Australia.

Think on the person you were as a child. Find a time in your childhood in which you felt you had a good sense of who you were. Record in writing, verbally or by some other creative representation, some spontaneous responses to the questions I have posed below. Remember to record your impressions freely, being sure not to edit your thoughts and feelings. This is for you, so record what you like and how you like.

- What were you like as a child, physically, mentally, emotionally and spiritually?
- Where did you live and what was it like?
- Who were the important people in your life?
- Why were these people important to you?
- What other influences were important in your childhood, such as other people, places and events?
- What were some of the 'rules for living' you learned from these people, places and events?

Now that you have created a cameo of yourself as a child, make some connections to your adult work life as a nurse or midwife, by responding freely to these questions:

- What were you like as a child, physically, mentally, emotionally and spiritually?
- Why did you want to become a nurse or midwife?
- Who were some of the important people in your life during your professional education?

- What is important in your practice and the ways you choose to work?
- What, if any, childhood 'rules for living' have been transferred into your adult work life as a practitioner?

From these descriptions, you may be able to see a little more clearly who you are as a person and a practitioner, and how you think nursing or midwifery should be practised according to your personal ideals.

You may find that the answers to some questions come quickly, while others need more time. Life is not always about positive memories either, and you may find that these questions bring up memories which may be tinged with sadness or some other emotion with which you have not dealt completely. This is a good point at which to make a comment about the depth of reflection. It is a good idea to reflect only to the level at which you are relatively comfortable. This does not mean that you avoid the challenges surrounding unfinished issues, but that you choose to look at them at the rate at which you are able to cope with them. This is not a process of deep psycho-analysis, as you need a skilled person to guide you in deep personal exploration. What is being encouraged here is your willingness to see yourself more clearly as a child so that you can connect yourself to the adult who is now a practitioner.

Your reflections

Using any of the strategies discussed earlier, spend some time recording your own story. When you have created a cameo of yourself as a child, it is a fairly simple step to connect yourself up to your adult work life as a practitioner. As always, respond as freely as you can to the questions listed in the previous reflector box.

From your descriptions you may now be able to see a little more clearly who you are as a person and a practitioner. They may tell you a little or a lot about how you think your life and work should be conducted according to some of your personal ideals. They may also serve to show you how values, beliefs and actions can slip somewhere in between the ideal expectations of childhood and the real experiences of adulthood. Keep your responses to this reflector, so that you can identify connections in the stories you are yet to record. It is amazing how ideas can fall into place when you take time to review them and put them into perspective.

DETERMINATION, COURAGE, A SENSE OF HUMOUR AND OTHER QUALITIES

After years of practising, teaching and researching reflection, I have come to the conclusion it takes some effort, which involves determination, courage and a sense of humour. Other qualities may be involved in reflection, but it seems to me that these requisites are essential. The reason I make this claim is that it is tempting to give up, to be afraid and to get far too serious about events which transpire as a result of a reflective life.

Determination

Determination is needed, for there may come a time when it all seems too difficult and you are tempted to return to an unreflective life, in which you do not have to be aware consciously of yourself, your work and the effects of the people and circumstances in your life. When the journey gets long and boring and you are feeling travel weary, you will need determination to keep on reflecting. It is similar to the resolve you need to maintain a commitment to yourself which requires effort, such as getting regular rest and exercise, or keeping regular purposeful contact with friends.

Courage

It takes courage to invest yourself in the depth of reflection which is needed to change procedures, interpersonal interactions and power relations at work. Timidity will not win the day when people start to question your motives, 'white-ant' your efforts, display open aggression to change, or block any progress you may be making. If I am painting a frightening picture at this point, it is because these events and more may happen. Added to the courage you need to face other people is that required to face yourself. Part of the reflective process is to identify patterns of thinking and behaving as a person and practitioner which may need adaptation. It is an oft-quoted cliché that the hardest journey you make is the one which leads home to yourself.

Humour

You may be thinking that reflection is sounding very complex and difficult because it takes determination, courage and more, but even though reflection needs to be approached seriously, it does not mean that you always have to take yourself seriously. For example, if a change in a ward procedure is fraught with technical errors, if practical reflection reveals a side of yourself you would rather not face, or if emancipatory reflection throws you into the front line as an advocate against oppressive structures, it can be made more bearable by a sense of humour. Nurses and midwives have the potential for 'black humour' which is based on insider knowledge, and this can be a great stress reliever in like-minded company. Being able to put situations into perspective by a light word, a grin or a well-placed joke may give you some respite from the enormity of it all. When I reflect on it, I manage and continue to work on some of the greatest challenges of my life through my sense of humour, because it lets me look differently at myself and other people.

Other qualities

Don't despair if you consider that you are deficient in determination, courage and humour as these qualities can be gained along the way and you will learn how to use them as you progress through the processes described in this book. You may also realise that there are many more qualities which can be nurtured through reflective practice that will fortify your life as a person and practitioner. This has been the case for many nurses and midwives who have used these processes before you, so take heart!

Here are some comments from midwives who were involved in some reflective practice research (Taylor et al. 1995). The first set of comments shows the amount of effort needed to reflect.

I found it quite daunting, actually, when I knew that I would be getting a call [from my critical friend] at seven o'clock, especially if you hadn't entered much in your journal. But, overall, I didn't worry if I felt tired and didn't really know what I was going to talk about, or if I hadn't entered anything in that particular week. But, generally, it was OK, not a big problem.

I've found it very time consuming for me with my baby and doing my degree as well, but I have used it effectively and it has certainly done some positive things for me too.

I think that the reflecting part (of my work) was an added pressure, and added things I had to think about. So I think it was just all the things together. I could have just sort of taken time out from something and all the other things would have been OK, but by adding one extra thing, that meant there was an extra pressure. I think it was worthwhile, because perhaps I would not have reflected on my work and my home life, and perhaps I wouldn't have noticed things weren't quite the same. And so, perhaps when I had finished that subject, I may not have tried to change anything . . .

On the positive side of the ledger, however, the midwives looked back at their achievements and were pleased they took the time and effort to reflect.

Yes, I think it's a really good process and it gives you a good laugh too that you're sort of serious about something and then a couple of months later you look back and think 'Well, I've achieved that.' You get really het up about something and then you look back a couple of months later and you think 'Oh well, that's working now. That's all better. That's one problem solved.' So it's a sense of achievement too.

I found the biggest benefit to me was that it was an outlet to talk about all the stresses in my life and probably come to grips with what was happening and probably get through it a bit more because I had sort of localised it and I found that quite helpful with group situations and studying and all the other things that are happening at the time.

[I've learned to] just stand up for myself more. I think

> I've found that. I think, reflecting back on this and looking at my practice, I have actually, these last few months . . . been standing up for myself more. Before, I'd sort of sometimes just go with the flow.

THE ROLE OF A CRITICAL FRIEND

Life can be all the easier because of the support of friends who provide congenial company and support you along the way. It is also good to have friends who are prepared to tell you some hard truths that you may not necessarily always like to hear. Critical friends support you and help you learn through challenging your attitudes and behaviour from time to time. When I think of my closest friends, they are the ones I trust and respect, and to whom I give permission to talk to me frankly if I am 'out of line' or failing to see something about myself and my situation which is apparent to them. This is the kind of friendship you need to nurture if you are serious about learning from your experiences.

This section is written for anyone who may become a critical friend. A critical friend is someone you trust and respect to assist you with your reflection. You may decide to swap from reflective practitioner to critical friend for someone you know, or you could use these suggestions and questions as another means of enhancing your own ability to reflect critically.

The role of your critical friend will be to listen to your clinical incidents and to assist you to make some sense of them. A critical friend gives guidance and support about your behaviours while being non-judgmental about you as a person. A critical friend needs to realise that he or she is not meant to be the person with the magical answers to every dilemma that you might raise, but rather that he or she is a person whose role is to encourage you to find the answers within yourself. By a well-timed question or a spontaneous supportive comment, a critical friend may provide the necessary support and stimulation for you to be the main 'sense-maker' of your reflections.

On the whole, critical friends listen more than they talk, and they avoid making early foreclosures on what they think might be the issues at hand. A critical friend will allow you to talk as much as you need to, in order to give a full description of the incident that occurred, so that there will be more substance to reflect on together. By allowing you to talk, he or she will allow you to come to your own awareness. She or he may ask a question here or there to clarify things and to point out inconsistencies in your thoughts and feelings if that becomes apparent.

Sometimes a critical friend may jot down notes of what seem to be the salient points as you speak, rather than interrupt the flow of your ideas. The critical friend may also take special interest in the words you use which suggest the emotional content of the story you are relating and the sense you made of your experiences then and since. If your story is very brief or it lacks sufficient details on which to reflect, your critical friend may encourage you to elaborate further.

A critical friend is willing to help you in a way which supports and challenges you so that you make the most sense out of your reflection. To do this well, there must be a sense of trust, respect and rapport and enough time and space to allow you to come to your own awareness. One of the ways in which you can be encouraged to go beyond your initial interpretation of your work issues is to explore the answers, if any, to questions which trigger reflection. Some reflective questions will be suggested in the next section.

Encouraging reflective questioning

Many questions for building descriptive stories are posed in the reflective processes in each of the sections in this book, but further questioning will assist you to stretch your imagination to consider hitherto unrealised possibilities. Whereas the suggestions that follow are by no means 'the definitive list,' they may be useful cues for you or your prospective critical friend to get you started on cycles of deeper reflection.

One of the most important parts of a reflective story is its emotional content, because if you can identify your feelings you can begin to reflect on why they are as they are and how to use them constructively. Therefore, if a critical friend can encourage you to express how you really felt about something that you have identified as problematic, contained within that disclosure may be some clues as to the nature and the effects of the problem itself and how it relates to you.

Questions to encourage reflection

Ask a colleague to tell you a story about a recent work incident in which they felt they made a positive difference to a person in their care. Explain that you will be listening with the intention of acting in the role of a critical friend. At appropriate intervals in the story, and according to the conventions of effective communication, ask any of the questions below in order to help your colleague provide a rich description of the incident.

* How were you feeling then?
* Why do you think you were feeling that way?
* How are you feeling about it now?
* Why do you think you are feeling that way?
* What sense did you have of . . . ?
* What was your spontaneous reaction to . . . ?

Other reflective questions are related to the content of the story and asked to draw out the features of the event so that a rich description can be generated. They include questions to keep the story flowing, such as:

* What happened then? When? Why? With whom?
* Can you tell me again about . . . ?

Other questions are attached to a restatement of what has been said previously and are useful for clarification and further elaboration. They include:

* You said before . . . Do you think that might be related to . . . ?
* What is the significance of . . . for you?
* Can you see any connections between this story and the one we discussed previously?
* It seems from what you said before that . . . What do you think of that?

Ask your colleague for any feedback on your role as

a critical friend. Ask what helped and what did not. Reflect on ways in which you can improve your role as a critical friend in future cases.

Some other kinds of questions are not easily listed because they come up as the conversation continues, but the chances are that they will emerge appropriately if your critical friend is attentive to the content and flow of what you are saying. Remember that not all questions have answers and some questions are worth asking for their rhetorical value. One of the benefits of asking questions in this process may be the realisation that it is OK to leave discussions open-ended and that quick-fix solutions are not always necessary or appropriate.

SUMMARY

In this chapter I described the basic essentials you need to prepare for reflection. I offered you some more information about reflective practice, and supplied you with a kitbag of strategies to help you on your way. I also suggested that you need determination, courage, a sense of humour and other qualities. A critical friend is also required, who will help by drawing your attention to points of interest along the way so that you can appreciate them more. I included some of the theoretical ideas about reflective practice, so that you could get a grasp on what matters most when you begin thinking about becoming a reflective practitioner.

4

Practitioners' reflections on their personal histories

In Chapter 3 I encouraged you to respond to a reflector about your personal history and how it has influenced you to become the person and practitioner you are now. Understanding yourself over time is important because it may help to 'fill in some gaps' in your appreciation of who you have become and why you think and act the way you do in your home and work life. On the assumption that people are complex individuals who are always learning about who they are, this process is very appropriate and helpful for thinking back systematically on childhood influences and how you have evolved your own rules for living that guide you now as a practitioner.

In Chapter 2 I introduced Esther, Michael and Carol. This chapter showcases what they wrote in response to the questions posed in Chapter 3 about childhood influences. I have not changed the way they wrote their accounts but they have checked the typed versions of their journal to add or delete any areas before their stories were included here.

ESTHER'S REFLECTIONS

My childhood was a mixed bag, like most, I guess. I spent a lot of time yearning for things my family either couldn't afford, or wouldn't allow. My father was rarely at home, worked too hard in oppressive conditions exerted by his elder brother and had difficulty in relating to myself and two older half sisters. He had been to both Africa/Middle East and New Guinea (as a commando behind enemy lines) in WWII, and, in reflection, had post-traumatic stress disorder which was never resolved as it was never recognised. I loved and envied him, the envy being for his freedom, his experiences and his strength. My mother was a loving presence, full of overt affection but very little else. To my lasting regret, I knew very little about her inner life and a part of her was very needy, dependent and sorrowful. She'd had a difficult life—wealthy parents (father imported carpets in NZ and Oz) who travelled a lot, boarding school at a young age, not achieving her goals of ballerina (she was accepted into Covent Garden, but chose to return to Australia) or nurse (left in second year to marry a doctor). Her first husband was apparently brilliant and came from a wealthy family—however, medicine wasn't enough—he studied law, couldn't cope and committed suicide (OD of barbiturates). Mum was left with two small girls at the end of the war, fortunately having supportive friends. Subsequently met my father after WWII and had a life without much money and love which faded over the years, to the point where Mum and Dad finally separated when I left home.

My sisters were kind strangers for most of my young life, as they were five and eight years older than me. They were a product of the war years while I was a baby boomer.

We lived in Cronulla, south of Sydney, close to

the sea. Our street was still dirt when I was young—memories of wet soil after the rain—the smell remains evocative to me—that, and playing in the raging gutters (no concrete) making dams. It always rained after the roads were graded. I spent half my life climbing trees, hiding my sandals when I went out and only putting them on when I came home. About three-quarters of our street was still bush.

I had a passion for cowboys (being one was my ambition) and I got many blood blisters practising swinging my father's old rifle around my fingers like Rifleman. I wanted a horse more than anything, but never had one. The next best thing was imagination, and myself and a group of friends had imaginary horses which we rode, groomed and cared for months, as if they were real.

I read constantly and can't remember learning to read—it seems to be something I've done forever. I had an eclectic taste and never seemed to be supervised regarding reading material. Consequently, I read a lot of adult stuff as well as children's books. Most of my childhood reading was adventure. As I grew older, I read vast amounts of books (mainly autobiographical) on the French Resistance Movement, classic Russian literature and some Tibetan Buddhism. I also had a passion for anything to do with Gypsies.

My passion for reading was mixed with an equal passion for the sea and surfing and these passions continue to the present day.

Important people in my life as a child were my mother for her love and my friends for their company. I have strong memories of my passionate interest in various subjects which just as quickly waned. I was, on reflection, not very disciplined and jumped from one interest to the next. I had loads of physical and intellectual ability which I squandered, to some extent. I fell in love with a boy from Canberra when I was fifteen—met on a school sport trip. Our relationship struggled through a few visits to each other's houses and lots of letters and finally died an impossible death when I left school early—halfway through Year 11—to 'go' nursing. My family's expectations for me were university. My best friend went to NZ as an exchange student and my restlessness drew me to quit school. The only way I was allowed was to start nursing—this was seen as respectable! Six months and I'd had enough. Instead of having the maturity and courage to admit that I was wrong, and go back to school, I got an office job where I met some interesting people. Two young women influenced my reading which I continued to do and I fell into a relationship aka Puberty Blues with a young man who surfed. The next couple of years culminated in a traditional 'white' wedding and travel, which was a driving force for me during the 70s—the overland trail, dope and the counter culture/hippie trip taught me about freedom, human rights and gave me the courage to defy my father regarding Vietnam and broader political issues. I came alive and realised that I needed to work altruistically.

One marriage over and another relationship began. I enrolled in nursing again, this time in the UK. Music, politics, Gough Whitlam and travel continued to be important as I battled to come to terms with patriarchal medicine and oppression in nursing.

Nursing has continued to be a love/hate

relationship for me. Love of the altruistic, compassion in the work, and hate for the bureaucratic, oppressive nature of the model in which I work.

However, tertiary education finally gave me a freedom to express myself, and my intellectual power meant that I could start exploring other ways of being in nursing, and without, in my personal life. Charles Sturt University and some of the faculty, Gail Hart, Tracy Brown and a sociology lecturer named Kerry became my mentors and I thrived. Reflective practice became second nature and my radicalism finally caught fire as I found nursing theory and research which supported previous gut feelings (perceptual awareness) regarding practice. Patricia Benner, Sandra Speedy, Anne Oakley and other feminist sociologists grounded my passion and fire so that I could now advocate for my patients, with the backing of nursing theory and research.

My personal approach to practice these days is generally one of confidence which is grounded in experience and knowledge—I try to make sure of that. My belief systems of honesty and courage, plus my Tibetan Buddhist practice of fearlessness and joy accompanied by compassion and empathy make for hard work every day in both personal and professional spheres. However, it's worth it, as I feel more alive now than ever before. I have a passion for my husband, my daughter and sons, my Buddhist philosophies, my commitment to making the health service egalitarian and life in general. Nursing/midwifery is a way of life for me it's not 'just a job'. I'm in it for the long haul, and while it may be frustrating and slow, I think globally and act locally, recognising small gains and changes for the better. I won't give up or give in. So, nursing/midwifery for me these days remains grounded in altruism, compassion, empathy, empowerment, equality and courage—without any of these attributes I couldn't practise with integrity.

So, important stuff in my life:

- equal rights
- Vietnam protests/radicalising my life
- Gough Whitlam
- literature
- music
- Chas, Esther, Oscar and Winston (husband and kids)
- feminism
- sociology
- Tibetan Buddhism
- love and compassion.

My 'rules for life', i.e. belief systems stem from both example and opposites of childhood experiences:

- unconditional love from my kids and my mother— example
- patriarchal behaviour from my father—opposite
- right wing politics from my father—opposite
- rigid, patriarchal religion—opposite
- love of dancing from my mother—example
- love of literature and travel from my mother—example
- opposition to oppression—myself
- equality, compassion and altruism—Chas and myself.

Are there any similarities between Esther's reflections about childhood influences and your own? How are your stories similar and different?

Esther wrote: 'Nursing has continued to be a love/hate relationship for me'. Can you identify influences in Esther's childhood which may have had love/hate aspects?

Note Esther's rules for life and you will see the influences she has chosen to exemplify or oppose in her adult life. Have you tended to adopt favourable aspects of people and situations as rules for your life and dismiss the less favourable? If yes, what are they? If not, why not, and how have you decided on your rules for life?

MICHAEL'S REFLECTIONS

Physically I was very slightly built as a child. I was very quiet, never spoke unless spoken to, well-mannered, considered the perfect student by teachers and received near-perfect grades. I've always been an anxious type of person but somehow manage for this never to show externally.

Religion played no part in my upbringing, whilst my Catholic friends think that this must be very refreshing not to carry guilt I think that growing up in the country brings about a sense of something similar.

As a child I often felt different from my peers but did not realise what was different until I was about fourteen and fell in love with my science teacher who was a male. The realisation that I was gay made a lot of things fit together. However, it did not avoid a lot of heartache associated with being a gay teenager in a country town.

At the age of 37 I still do not feel fully accepted by my family. It is more a tolerance than acceptance given that my father-in-law refuses to acknowledge I exist. I suppose I should be grateful. I would like total acceptance from my family but feel this is probably asking a lot of people who believe Pauline Hanson is a saint.

My father was a school teacher in country schools and as such we shifted several times during my schooling. I always found settling into new schools difficult, trying to establish new friends in small conservative communities who saw you as an outsider. My father was also my school teacher in grades 5–6 which made it very difficult to have a relaxed relationship.

Important people in my childhood were: My mother—who I could strangle for her conservative country values at times but who stuck by her family in what I suspect was a very unfulfilling marriage for her because it was the right thing to do. This was not really evident until she remarried in her late 50s and has become a far happier and content person. My mother has a great sense of humour which is very black at times it is something we share in common.

My mother had a very close friend, Irene. She was the only true close friend my mother ever had. They went everywhere together. Irene's life had not been easy, she had lost a son in an MCA on Christmas Eve, a few years later her house burned down and all belongings and photos of her son were destroyed. Irene was scarred emotionally and physically from this accident but made the most of every opportunity given to her. Lessons I learned from Irene are to speak your mind, good humour and making every day count.

My Aunty Olga—Olga was a close relative as two sisters married two brothers and Olga was my Mum's closest sister. Olga was the first person to ever accept me as a gay teenager and show me unconditional love. I think this is the most important lesson I received from Olga and generally I think I tolerate and accept all people well. We all have our days though.

Aunty Myrtle—My Mum's great aunt. My substitute grandmother as my grandmother died giving birth to child number eleven. Aunty Myrtle was a generous person who had a great love of travel and making the most of every opportunity. Bordering on eccentric by the time she died I loved the things she did like photocopying extras of wedding invitations she received and sending them on to people she thought should go too. From my Aunty Myrtle I developed my love for travel and always being willing to explore wider horizons.

Something already stands out as I look back at my childhood and that is that all the people who influenced my childhood are women. Is this because I'm gay or did this cause me to be gay? Who cares, if the latter is the case then I have even more to thank them for because I would never change my sexuality.

My father's influence in my childhood is more a negative than a positive. I remember him as a drinker who made us wait outside hotels for him and having to help him to the car when he was legless. I don't recall this as being often but enough to make a lasting impression through to my adulthood.

Places: My growing up was along the Murray River and still to this day I always feel like I'm home when I am near the Murray. I find it a very peaceful and relaxing place to be.

Lessons from my childhood: I guess the main lesson is about a sense of family and as a result family is still very important to me. I find it amusing as I struggle for acceptance from the family that in a time of crisis I am the one who will be called upon. I suspect this is true of a lot of nurses because we think clearly whilst others around are floundering.

Rules: I don't recall any great restrictions or rules in my childhood. My brother and I often received advice from our parents which we disregarded and later regretted disregarding it. We have always been given the opportunity to learn from mistakes and this is alive and well in my nursing practice.

Nursing: Nursing was something I was talked into by some friends, not unusual for a male as I don't imagine many young boys choose nursing as what they want to do when they grow up. My only experience of hospitals was as a three-year-old having my tonsils removed. It is a recollection which is vivid to me being left alone with all those strangers.

My father was perhaps the most important influence during my education and training. Diagnosed with lung cancer in my first year of training I was able to experience being the family of a patient first hand. I was able to observe so much and take mental notes of things I vowed I would never do to patients or their families. In my father's terminal stage I was aware of how distant nurses were, obviously keeping to themselves. To keep it all in perspective, these nurses were also my colleagues and I was rostered to work in the ward where he died so it was a difficult situation for everybody. The night nurse on duty was renowned for falling asleep on duty so I used to go home wondering if my father required something would somebody be there. From this I made sure that no one who is a relative would ever be doubtful about my nursing care or standard of practice. When my father died the two days of compassionate leave were taken up by weekend days and on the Monday I had to negotiate with the DON to take leave without pay to go to my father's funeral. I promised myself that as a manager I would be far more sympathetic with staff than anything that had been my experience at this time.

Irene, my Mum's friend, had completed three years of nursing training but failed her final exams so never got to practice. She helped me study and kept me motivated as things deteriorated at home during the first year of my training. The night before my exams at the end of second year she arrested and died at 49 years of age. Knowing what it would have meant to her to be able to practise as a nurse made me determined to finish my nursing at a time when it would have been far easier to walk away.

A brief mention to one of the educators in the School of Nursing at the time of my training. Our friendship extended back to when I was a bank teller and would see her when she came into the bank. She was a good friend who always helped you keep things in perspective. Most of all she was the one who gave students of nursing a sense of future when her colleagues were struggling to hold onto the past.

The good humour (as black as you could imagine) required to lighten the day-to-day load was provided by Judy K. Judy and I went through each ward and specialty area together, we holidayed together. I would have been her bridesmaid but we didn't think the country was ready for that yet.

My personal approach to practice: I guess the

major way to describe my approach to practice is sharing—making patients part of the decision-making process regarding their care. I always discuss what I would see as a reasonable plan for the day but am happy to negotiate a different plan if it is more suitable to the patient.

I love to listen to patients telling me their story, taking the time to find out about life outside a hospital room so that you piece together the whole picture.

The major thing I strive for is a sense of fun and enjoyment in my work. When a job ceases to be enjoyable I leave to find something else. That's why after fifteen years of nursing I am nine years away from long service.

I believe my absolute strength is in making my colleagues aware of how valuable they are as clinicians by giving them every bit of positive feedback I can. I believe in the role of the nurse in the healing process and want nurses around me to feel that they and their work is an important part of the healing process.

The main 'rule for living' taken from my childhood and education which I have transferred into my nursing practice is my acceptance of patients. I believe I am largely non-judgmental when dealing with patients. When I feel myself being pushed to the limits as some patients can do, my sense of humour kicks in and generally I manage to see a black side to situations that would drive anybody else to distraction. The real bonus to this is (I jest!) that every time there is a 'difficult' patient or situation happening I am always called upon as I will remain cool in most situations.

I feel I am at risk of sounding greater than Flo herself with what I have described to you so I must *tell you the things that bring out the worst in me in my practice.*

I am absolutely intolerant of laziness or people who make it clear (in their statements and by their practice) that they are only in nursing for the money or to see the children through private school, etc. When a patient is compromised by nursing practice that is borne out of laziness or ignorance then you see me at my absolute worst.

Michael wrote: 'The main 'rule for living' taken from my childhood and education which I have transferred into my nursing practice is my acceptance of patients.'

As you read through Michael's personal history, ask yourself why acceptance is important to him.

To what extent is acceptance of patients important to you?

What did you write about your main rule for living? Why is it important for you?

Think of questions you would ask Michael if you could act in the role of his critical friend to explore any of the issues he raises in his personal history. If you refer to Chapter 3 you will see the types if questions you could ask.

CAROL'S REFLECTIONS

Born in a big city of parents alone and from the country themselves. After moving a few times with happy times and other brothers and sisters born into the family. At CH started school and began a school career of quiet achievement. Picked on by some of the 'bad boys' occasionally.

Stole a bit of money from Mum's purse to make myself look bigger in front of my friends. We didn't get any money from Mum and Dad, they started after the stealing but that soon faded.

Busy childhood really between school, Girl Guides, tennis, then working on the weekend and Sunday School.

I learned a lot in those days. I loved camping and learning and projects and achieved high in Girl Guides—Queens Guide and then Queens Scout in Scouts/Venturers. The values instilled in us then are still very much a pert of my life now, e.g. respect for others, doing good turns, honesty, loyalty, comradeship, adventure.

A quiet achiever, not the most intelligent but in high classes at school. Character quiet, worked long hours on projects, little help from parents but got on with life.

Values from parents to work hard, finish things, be careful to dress neatly, clothes ironed and shoes polished even though they may not be new. Dad in the Navy. I wasn't the son he wanted but he did have a son who went into the Navy and followed in his footsteps in more ways than one. Dad was encouraging, we discussed politics, my projects, he took us places to camps, but we certainly didn't get any extras. Mum worked, she sewed for us too. I always wore what she made and didn't argue with that. The clothes she chose were sometimes old fashioned but I was grateful and didn't complain.

I was, and still am, a bit on the plump side, my brothers and sisters all taller and slimmer than I. But I had a few more brains. The usual sibling rivalry between us but the moment anyone picked on a sibling we were there in defence and support of each other and this still happens in our adult life. Loyalty is a good thing I learned. In most of the places I worked loyalty was good but medicolegal 'cover thy butt' work practices and selfish people I work with destroy loyalty, but you could say that is the way the system is now.

My parents split when I was thirteen, then back together soon afterward and then left again—selfish shouting and yelling. There was nothing I could do about it. I don't think I ever blamed myself. But I did see a video once of four children's reaction to divorce whilst I was working at Karitane dealing with dysfunctional families. The video showed how these four kids responded and it gave me insight into the way us four reacted. One was angry and loud, another withdrew and moved so we didn't know his whereabouts (I find this pathetic behaviour and totally selfish), another just got on with life. No real rebellion, no drugs, etc.

I left home and went to Sydney to do my nurse's training. I got into all the nursing schools, even in my home town but still wanted to go to the big city. I was in a big nursing school and was a bit homesick coming home on the bus on a twelve-hour ride. I hated it after a while. My family practically never came to Sydney and I rang them, they never rang me. Mum eventually came to my graduation actually she came to three of my graduations so that's not bad out of five. When my younger sister came to

Sydney and Mum had a new husband she came more often to Sydney to see my sister but it didn't really matter then, I was past being homesick and quite established in Sydney.

Nursing—I struggled with a number of things. The routines of the wards, the forcefulness of the sisters. We had it good really, we were in an era of nursing coming out. We didn't have to 'live in'. We got rid of hats in my second year as a student. We could talk to the sisters and be friends with senior nurses and called the supervisors by their first name. Our wages doubled in no time and we seemed always to be having a protest march up the main street of Sydney, bashing on bed pans, 'Don't get sick you won't get a bed!!' I loved it, it was a time for action, nurses standing united and fighting for a cause together. Not like nowadays, stabbing each other in the back, stepping over colleagues to get better jobs or the top ones, stealing other people's ideas without acknowledgment.

I was quite shy, did as I was told. My first year they told me I wasn't suited and could leave if I liked—was there anything else I was interested in or would I like a second chance? I took the second chance but they also didn't help me at all, you are on your own. Nothing has changed much in nursing. It is still teach yourself and if you are having difficulties there isn't much support.

After my training I did the usual 'Europe' overseas jaunt for nine and a half months. Went over with two friends and we were going to travel round but they wanted to stay and my parents broke up again for the second and last time. I was still shy but easily mixed with the other quiet ones (when I look back and we were probably the majority) it always reminds me of that movie Revenge of the Nerds. The majority of school and the world are 'nerds' so why should the short, plumpy, not so beautiful, glasses-wearing people worry about it so much we are in the majority.

Advertising has done a disservice to the world's population and to people's self-esteem—if we aren't skinny, tall and beautiful then we aren't worth as much.

As I am older and much more secure as a person and I know I am worthwhile as a person, then one of my biggest challenges in life is to encourage women, especially those I work with as midwives and patients that they are worthwhile. Empower them with increased self-esteem as much as possible.

I always want to do the best with my clients, encourage them with their mothercraft skills and build up their self-esteem. My philosophy at present: 'If we have a healthy, happy mother then the baby will be fine.' I am mother-focused and even to the point of not liking babies, they are so boring they don't 'do' anything.

Who I was as a child? Quiet but with a bit of a temper. Comfortable in my home environment. I felt secure, my parents were there most of the time when we needed them. My mother had a job with split shifts which meant she was home when we got home from school we could chat and tell her about things we did that day and then we could have tea and get on with other things. We looked after each other when I was twelve. Four of us and a real power thing, where I was the boss because I was the oldest but a real comradeship as well and this support and comradeship continue till present times.

Very busy with projects. I liked reading I was a bit slow and meticulous with reading and study. I couldn't skim things through or skip chapters—perhaps a thoroughness. I am still like this, but getting a bit more game and trying to work smarter not harder. I am now studying for a Masters and there is so much to wade through some material has to be skipped, not enough time.

Physically plump sporty but not the fastest or best. Team sports fairly good. Good technically cricket, soccer, not scared or timid.

Emotionally I think fairly stable very quiet, not sure of myself a lot and still am now thinking I am not as good as the other person but yet at the same time an achiever. Queens Guide, Queens Scout, teaching Sunday School, playing tennis, working at a fruit and vegetable shop on the weekends, reading studying. I must have had drive and enthusiasm.

Loved craft, crocheting and any other tapestry, macrame. My sister did the more way out stuff— pottery and buys craft things and doesn't use them again. My Mum was a big influence, she sewed, didn't knit but encouraged us with our handicrafts, etc., brought up working in the gardens.

Where did we live? Can't remember the early years before school, only snippets we moved. Born in Newcastle; Tamworth where K and G were born, then Coffs. I started school then to L and M was born. A rented house with boys that were our own age and I remember they used to touch in private places but we moved from there so we weren't there long. Our new house Mum and Dad built and near to school. We were comfortable.

Important people were my Sunday School teacher. She would treat us all like we were important, called us 'people' rather than kids or anything else. She was significant. My parents and teachers, yeah, they were there. My friends at school fairly significant, we used to have discussions and major debates, I like that and I think I still like a good discussion and its amazing in certain circles there is always a person to discuss something with.

Rules for living: Dad—be clean and neat, value things and look after them because you can't just replace things. I remember he was always encouraging, having these discussions. Work hard.

Mum showed us examples of persevering no matter where the chips were even if they were down. When the family split she was encouraged by a Real Estate man (her uncle) to buy the other side of the house, so financially, the divorce was good. One house splits, one person buys the other half getting a whole and the other with his deposit buys another house with a mortgage and eventually pays that off so from one house now becomes two.

The dirty laundry really came a few years after their divorce. Another woman came into my father's life in 1985–86. She was very controlling, a right bitch in fact. My father from a confident all knowing man became a mouse controlled by this woman. Back to court to take the other half of Mum's house after she paid for it (there was a stamp missing off some legal papers). What a greedy bastard, he had one half and now wanted the other. The woman had hassled her previous husband too and now she was pushing Dad.

Three years court case. In the end Dad lost and

had to pay maintenance in a lump sum and so that paid Mum's legal fees. Interesting behaviour on my mother's part. She used to talk about it all the time, exaggerate a bit perhaps for sympathy perhaps crying out for someone to listen and help her somehow. I think that I do this now. I have had difficulty at work for a while and I can see no way out so I talk to people and sometimes exaggerate (not much though) just so someone will help me but no one does, everyone looks after themselves.

When the second court case came I thought my mother would lay down and die, but to my surprise she didn't, she had friends and she found out things the solicitor could not. I saw an empowered woman and she fought and she won.

My father has nothing to do with us now and he says he has a new family. What a pathetic man who lets a woman dominate him.

Why did I want to become a practitioner? I wanted to be a physio, I can't really remember why. I applied to uni and as a nurse to the local and big Sydney hospitals. I got into all of them and also uni in Wagga to be a nurse (they only did nursing at uni in a couple of places then). So I chose Sydney. I wanted to experience life more. I could have stayed at home and gone training locally but didn't. It was a good decision, those who train at this hospital have a particular mentality very narrow and vindictive some of them. Is that the person or the hospital, who knows?

My training years I talked about in first few pages. Active with union marches to improve the patients lot.

Active with church activity. I had a choice to have friends who went to the pub or to church. I would have been a great addict because when I get into something it is full on. I thank God I went to church and found another family who were supportive for years. Also I became a Cub Leader (Boy Scouts). We did heaps of stuff over the four years, very busy!

I once thought about it. I had a bit of a temper at times just like my father. I obviously wanted to be like him but I sat back one day and looked at his behaviour. His temper really only got him trouble or people didn't like him because he thought he was always right. So I decided there is only a certain amount of energy, I could use it in anger or I could channel it into something constructive. So I did, I put all my energy into heaps of things. Anger doesn't solve problems.

Some of the educators were significant. Some were pathetic, others very inspiring. One woman stands out, she was a science teacher and we were all waiting one morning for the science lab, we were all sitting on the ground. She was chatting and said 'at the end of your training one out of four of you will be gay'. I thought this was an interesting thing to say to a bunch of impressionable first years, half of which came from the country and believed everything the tutors told us.

I met her again ten years ago when I was doing my conversion to the degree. She was doing her PhD then and still as gay as ever but an excellent lecturer.

The gay influence over the years is interesting. It was very subtle at first. PA had heaps but none really impacted on me then. At Paddo there were heaps, at one stage there was so many I had to ask myself was I one as well and after thinking about it realised I liked men too much so I wasn't gay. Then a big blow was a good friend, we used to go camping and hiking, and she all of a sudden didn't have anything to do with me as she had turned gay. I was very upset not because she was gay but because she had rejected our friendship. Now I have an answer to whingeing gays who think 'normals' are victimising them, but I think it is a reverse victimisation—they reject me because I am normal.

Other influences—the church we had a lot of Asian students and I was very lucky to be accepted as one of them even given my own Chinese name, so when I came across foreigners in the wards I could even greet them in Chinese asking 'how are you going?' and an immediate bond even though I couldn't speak any more except asking for the bill. Their cultural beliefs I got to know, like instead of getting a jug of ice water when they were in labour, getting a jug of hot water and their custom not to wash afterward. Something to do with the Yin and Yang.

I have now travelled to a lot of places in Asia, mainly staying with friends. I go overseas every year. The people at work greet me with where are you going now? I usually have a holiday planned. They ask where do I get the time but I can answer I get the same time allocated as everyone and get the same wage so it just depends on your organisational skills and your determination and perhaps opportunity.

I think my enthusiasm for life, travel and study, etc. has challenged many I work with to strive for more in life. It has been to my detriment at times. My personality of being shy but lashing out at times at unjust or frustrating situations is not tolerated easily by the status quo. I am working on my reactions though.

My personal approach to practice? Back in the

dim dark ages we used to spin the story of why we wanted to become nurses and the usual statement 'we wanted to help people'. We all laugh but that was the line that we used.

The discriminating hospitals were just as bad. North Shore's question was 'what does your father do?'

A lot of women went into nursing because of the fact we got paid and had a place to live—'Menopause Mansion'.

My practice back then was help the patients, do the washes, do the practical work. A lot of task allocation, but that stopped not long after I started. We had pay rises, got rid of hats and patient allocation came in so the hierarchy became squashed and we could even talk to the sisters and 'white shoe syndrome' was not a big thing.

The other influence was the college nurses. I worked with some very early in the piece. I was nearly one myself. I had a fascination with them. They knew the theory and after a bit of practice also caught up with us experts who had the practical experience. But then I noticed they passed the hospital training people. They had more theory behind them and in the long run they were perhaps 'better'. So the decision was to go along with so many other hassling and putting them down or befriend them. It was a good decision so early on in my career.

They are the same as we were. Some are born nurses; others, just like in the hospital system, shouldn't be there. At least they left earlier from the college because they didn't have the money incentive to stay like the hospital apprenticeship system.

I had difficulties with the basics. There was always too much to do and not enough time. I was perhaps a bit lazy. But I also wanted to be with the patients—talking to them, treating them like normal people, crying with them if they were sad. We saw numerous deaths which was fairly traumatic and the only support we got was from our fellow nurses.

Back to the question—describe my personal approach to practice. Do the work, get it done, do as I was told—General. On to midwifery.

Just before I got into midwifery I spent nine months in Europe travelling and then three months in PNG which changed my philosophical practice completely. Maybe I grew up a bit more and saw what else nurses could do. Also I wanted to be a missionary who worked in Africa or PNG. In PNG they were either dead or dying. None of this back rub shit. These babies and kids were dying because of lack of antibiotics. I thought back to all the waste we had in the hospitals in Australia.

In PNG the sisters were really the doctors. They were ordering drugs, diagnosing, doing forceps and ventoses. They had to make the decision often to ship the woman out who had already walked for three days and had been in labour two days before that.

The prem babies were born up there the same as here but they had no humidicribs. What did they do?? All these things and heaps more thinking. I came back and started midwifery training at Paddington.

Great hospital, huge, I loved the anonymity of it all. I didn't know the patients and they never saw you again mostly. I liked the privacy but I had my own group of friends. Life was busy.

I continually asked many questions like 'what will the doctor do when he gets here?' to be told 'wait till he gets here' and then 'do as he says'. But I continued to question and anticipate management.

My father got remarried ten days before my mid final. I failed, but so did 50 per cent of our class. So we just sat it again in six months and passed.

After three and a half years at Paddington I went to the Birth Centre to work. I learned a philosophy of spiritual midwifery far from the medical model. To empower a woman to birth and not to be delivered. To allow them to have control over their own situation, their own decisions and the consequences. One midwife said to me after I had asked her to teach me something, 'Let the women teach you. Ask them what they are feeling and going through.' Learn from them!!!!

I learned to give the women control and the power of the female body was awesome. I saw women stop and start labours. One significant birth was in the shower and a multigravida was going so much slower than normal. Then as she was pushing and the head came out she said to the husband 'is it normal, is it normal?' He said 'yes' and then the baby shot out so quickly. She said later she was too scared to have the baby because a doctor in the Antenatal Clinic said there was something wrong with the baby's head and she had been thinking about this and was so scared to deliver an abnormal baby. But he was normal.

Wow, the power of the psyche. The power that the words we say have and wow the power to stop and start labours that medicine has been unable to do ever!!

Next—my time at Karitane Mothercraft Hospital basically carried on from the Birth Centre philosophy.

In the Early Childhood Centre the families had to take the child home so I gave the power to the women. Some could handle it, some couldn't. Some liked the previous sister who took control and told them what to do. I didn't do this. We worked as a team mostly. We worked plans out together and often I would ask 'what would you like to do?'

The women were empowered and I had a reputation and gained many women, usually difficult ones, who then came voluntarily to the clinic. We worked together. They opened up more and told me things that they had done like sneak some chocolate over Easter and when I asked did the kid play up they said no and so the old wives tale of not being able to eat chocolate when you breastfeed was bunkum.

My professional support was poor. I rang my boss to consult with her and she said network in the community. But where? I didn't know where. Then one of my confidantes was one of the formula reps, she was an ex-social worker so when she came she dumped the formula in the corner and I would consult about strategies with my difficult cases. I needed support too!!!!!!

Some of the more problem ones had their tricks. They would come just before closing at lunch time and dump their 'stuff'. They knew I would listen but I also had to eat and had a toaster and had stuff in the fridge to put on it and one woman was shocked when I asked her to join me and she said she didn't think clinic sisters ate, let alone with 'the clients'.

I left the clinic. To be young and single and having a lot of dumping done on me it was getting quite heavy. Maybe my own support systems weren't good enough to cope and I probably took on myself too many of the women's problems.

But I went on to an Educator position. Lecturing at the University of Western Sydney in the Karitane course and writing two modules for the course. A great experience.

My sister said the women in the clinic will survive without me. I moved on for myself.

Summary now after eighteen years as a nurse and midwife.

Give the control to the women, educate them, empower them. Some can't handle it so just support them along. The medical model has many holes in it, midwifery proves it. There is no answer to many of the questions. But to survive in life we must encourage the women. If I can make even the slightest difference in someone's life then my practice is worthwhile.

In this story, Carol shared many of her thoughts, feelings and values about what matters most to her in her adult life and how she has evolved to the person and practitioner she is today. Carol's willingness to write freely enhances this story as it gives her much 'food for thought' should she want to review it in light of new awareness. This is the case with all reflection—that it is amenable to change based on renewed awareness.

Identify some of the values Carol uses as a practitioner.

In her summary, Carol asserted her intention in midwifery to assist women. Trace the influences which may have had a bearing on her present intention to empower women through her midwifery practice.

PLEASE NOTE

Esther, Michael and Carol have offered generously some reflections on their childhood influences and we have been treated to some of their innermost thoughts. When you undertake this exercise it may take you back to many memories you have not visited for some time and with which you may feel involved emotionally. It is important to reflect only at the levels with which you are prepared to deal. It cannot be stressed enough that these forms of reflection are not intended to be at deep psychoanalytical levels, but rather that they are from the levels with which you are willing and ready to face. In other words, you may experience emotion such as laughter and tears, but it is my intention that you will be able to face your memories beneficially, and not be overwhelmed or paralysed psychologically by them. Therefore, ensure that you deal with what you can, at the rate which suits you.

SUMMARY

In this chapter Esther, Michael and Carol shared their responses to a reflector posed in Chapter 3 about their personal histories to show how they have been influenced to become the people and practitioners they are now. Reviewing where you have been tells you where you are now and raises possibilities for where you might go next with reflection.

5

The value of reflection

REFLECTION IS VALUABLE FOR ALL PRACTITIONERS

Practitioners exercise a profession and are involved in a discernible practice. Professionals achieve their status if they have the basic requisites of belonging to a professional group. Although most of the literature on professions is dated, some of it is worth reviewing, because it may show you why some nurses and midwives are still 'fighting over old ground'.

The features of practice professions

Professionalisation is the process through which an occupation becomes a profession. The ways in which an occupation transforms itself into a profession vary, but are generally considered to entail a strong level of commitment, a long and disciplined educational process, a unique body of knowledge and skill, discretionary authority and judgment, active and cohesive professional organisation, and acknowledged social worth and contribution.

Goode (1966, in Freidson 1970) describes professions according to two core characteristics: 'a prolonged specialised training in a body of abstract knowledge' and 'a collectivity or service orientation', with autonomy for professional standards and education, licensing, legislation and freedom from lay evaluation and control. Freidson (1970), however, argues that the only truly important and uniform criterion for distinguishing professions from other occupations is the fact of autonomy—a position of legitimate control over work (1970: 82). He adds that professionalisation often requires the support of powerful groups within the social structure. This being so, one can only wonder at the degree of support nursing and midwifery could realistically expect from medicine, given that their ascendancy might mean less subservience to medicine.

The professionalisation of an occupation is, to some extent, at the expense of the community. Freidson (1970: 18) describes a profession primarily as 'a special status in the division of labour supported by official and sometimes public belief that it is worthy of such status'. He also claims that a 'profession's service orientation is a public imputation it has successfully won in a process by which its leaders have persuaded society to grant and support its autonomy' (1970: 8). In this sense, a profession's autonomy is won at the considerable expense of the members of a community in that the specialised knowledge it generates and owns becomes a means of domination in which a 'special status in the division of labour [is] supported by official and sometimes public belief that it is worthy of such status' (1970: 187).

In relation to the issues of domination of people by professions in complex civilisations in which people create knowledge, laws, morals and procedures, Freidson (1970) claims:

> the official social order is politically and culturally dominant, reflecting the values and knowledge of the dominant classes of the society. It is not necessarily hostile to the values of everyday life, but it is nonetheless imposed on everyday life, and its imposition is supported by organised political, economic and normative forces. (1970: 30)
>
> . . . And when experts constitute a profession, their knowledge and values become part of the official order which however enlightened, liberal and benevolent, is nonetheless imposed on the everyday world of the layman [sic]. (1970: 303)
>
> . . . Furthermore, on an everyday basis they serve as gatekeepers to special resources . . . that cannot be used without permission. Thus the behaviour of the physician and others in

the field of health constitutes the objectification, the empirical embodiment of certain dominant values in a society. (1970: 304)

The power and privilege afforded to professionals by society also carry responsibilities. The professional is expected to behave in an appropriate manner, often in culturally proper and detached ways, distancing the professional emotionally and intellectually from clients. Freidson (1970: 336–37) expresses the separation of professionals from clients and the claim that medicine has taken responsibility for moral decisions as an instrument of social control:

> The relation of the expert to modern society seems in fact to be one of the central problems of our time, for at its heart lie the issues of democracy and freedom and of the degree to which ordinary men [sic] can shape the character of their own lives. The more decisions are made by experts, the less they can be made by laymen [sic] . . . expertise is more and more in danger of being used as a mask for privilege and power rather than, as it claims, as a mode of advancing the public interest. (1970: 337)

Of practitioners, Freidson (1970) writes:

> First, the aim of the practitioner is not knowledge but action . . .
>   Second, the practitioner is likely to believe in what he [sic] is doing in order to practice. (1970: 168)
>   . . . But unlike other workers, the professional clinician's belief in his [sic] functionally diffuse wisdom is reinforced strongly by the respectful receipt of his [sic] opinions by a lay world that does not discriminate between what is functionally specific to his [sic] training and what is not. (1970: 171)

The effect of society's deference to a professional clinician's wisdom and skill is control, in the sense of providing services clients do not or may not want, practising paid caring services as a matter of routine, decreasing interference and increasing convenience for the practitioner, and the generation of better procedures as clinicians become more skilful. The institutional treatment of illness has the effect of isolating patients from the lay community, by rationing contact with the lay community and decreasing information to people generally (Freidson 1970).

Discuss the idea with colleagues that the effect of society's deference to a professional clinician's wisdom and skill is control. Do you think that this is true of medical practitioners? Why?

Do you think that nurses and midwives exercise control over their clients by virtue of the services they provide? Why?

In responding to this reflector, it may help to identify clinical situations in which you have witnessed controlling behaviours by doctors or nurses.

Regardless of the professional group affiliation, it becomes apparent that the rights and responsibilities of practice professionals are immense and that the whole area is intensely political. Added to this are the complexities of practice settings and relatively unexpected outcomes of courses of treatment and choices for action. Therefore, practitioners need some kind of systematic process for reviewing their work practices to determine effectiveness in light of their work constraints. This is the basis of reflective practice and the processes described in this book.

Are nursing and midwifery professions?

The debate has raged for some time as to whether nursing and midwifery are professions, and to date the answers seem to be 'Yes', 'No' and 'Maybe'. Merton (1957) claims that to reach the pinnacle of the professional hierarchy and stay in place requires the continuation of service functions and associated roles. This depends on monopolisation of the direct and related functions of the occupation and high social class for both the occupation and its members.

In the 1980s there was a spirited debate as to the professional status or otherwise of nursing and midwifery and, to some extent, the issue has been left unresolved. Crowder (1985) reviewed the criteria for a profession as stated by eleven theorists and found that, among the 41 characteristics generated, nursing fared quite well, except in the areas of autonomy and control.

If autonomy over work is the mark of a profession, are

nursing and midwifery professions if they are reliant on 'doctor's orders'? Freidson (1970: 69) focuses on nursing and argues that it is subject to another occupation and thus is not a profession:

> An aggressive occupation like nursing can have its own schools for training, can control licensing boards in many instances, and can have its own 'service' in hospital, in this way giving the appearance of formal, state-supported, and departmental autonomy, but the work which its members perform remains subject to the order of another occupation.

Whether nursing and midwifery have control in terms of their relations with doctors and other health professionals is a moot point; however, nursing and midwifery can be seen as having control in some crucial areas. For example, Freidson (1970: 123) sees nurses as having control in respect to patients, deducing that, 'from the accumulation of studies of interaction on the ward, a number of patient attributes seem to have important bearing on what techniques of control can be exercised by staff members seeking to order their work'.

In a standard pro-medical text, Robinson (1978) attempts to dilute Freidson's assertive stance on professions, claiming that the two core characteristics of professions are a prolonged specialised training in a body of abstract thought and a collectivity or service orientation. Of these two traits, Goode (1966 in Freidson 1970: 135) says that an occupation may 'rank high on one but low on another. Thus nursing ranks high on the variable of service orientation but has been unable to demonstrate that its training is more than low-level medical evaluation.'

Write and discuss your views on whether you think nursing and midwifery are professions. Share these ideas with colleagues and canvas their opinions. Note points of difference in their positions—that is, the ways in which they disagree with each other. Explore with them the extent to which they think that nursing and midwifery are medically dominated occupations, and see if they connect this issue with failure to achieve professional status.

Speedy (1987) argues that the path to professionalisation must include recognition by nurses (and midwives) that they are oppressed groups, and that they need to act to rectify this. One of the main sources of oppression is medical dominance of nursing and midwifery. Kelly (1985) questiones the orthodox structure of health care delivery, reporting a challenge to physicians as the sole primary health care providers, focusing on legal issues raised against nurse practitioner services: licensing restrictions, third-party reimbursement policies, and denial of access to medical facilities and physician back-up services.

It should be noted that there have been advances in nurses' and midwives' autonomy as practitioners. For example, in 1998 important legislation passed through the New South Wales Parliament to approve the registration of Nurse Practitioners who can act autonomously in private practice as professionals. Also, midwifery is claiming its professional status through direct entry programs of education; private practice agreements now allow hospital visits for childbirth, and provide medical and allied support services for the care of women through the entire pregnancy, labour, delivery and postnatal periods.

REFLECTION IS VALUABLE FOR NURSES AND MIDWIVES

The assumption made in this book is that nurses and midwives are professional practitioners by virtue of their practice knowledge and skills. Reflection is valuable for nurses and midwives because it gives them the means whereby they can track their way systematically through practice issues to arrive at new insights and the potential for improvement and change. People who become nurses and midwives may start out with the usual motives of caring for people or, more recently, of finding and keeping meaningful employment. Experienced practitioners realise invariably that there is more to nursing and midwifery than they first thought. Fanciful ideals of helping people can be tested in the grim realities and challenges of practice. Personal rules for living need to be stretched to accommodate unexpected human situations. Practice may not turn out to be what it first seemed, and nurses and midwives may struggle to hold on to the ideals of why they wanted to practise in the first place. In the face of these personal and professional dilemmas, reflection is a valuable source of stability in an otherwise changing and unpredictable world of work.

Although there is value in being a reflective practitioner, you should realise that reflective practice is not without its critics. For example, I have argued that nursing and midwifery are complex work contexts and almost like battlefields, and that it is foolhardy for teachers to encourage clinicians to reflect on and try to change their practice in settings unsupported by collective political action (Taylor 1997). Also, various authors have questioned the scope and depth of reflective processes (Clarke et al. 1996; Clinton 1998). Even so, these arguments amount to no more than cautionary notes to the claims about the value of reflective practice. The position I take in this book is to assume that the creation of a systematic and thoughtful approach to practice is a good beginning for making positive differences in your life and work. Whereas it might not solve all your problems and offer you all the answers you require to your practice dilemmas, such processes help you to face the complexities of your practice experiences.

Some testimonies from previous research

With Virginia King and Julia Stewart, I undertook some research (Taylor et al. 1995) with midwives to guide them in reflective processes and to monitor their responses. The study involved ten self-selected midwives, who were enrolled in a Bachelor of Health Science (Nursing) Midwifery unit. The midwives were given a learning package about reflective processes, they kept reflective logbooks, and they had weekly phonecall contact with a designated facilitator. A teleconference at end of the eight-week research period evaluated the experience. The information collected was interpreted at individual and collective levels. Practitioners were encouraged to interpret and share their own practice experiences throughout the process. Transcripts of audiotaped conversations and facilitators' notes were analysed by manual thematic analysis, for themes which emerged as indicative of the value of the reflective practice experience.

Without exception, participants acknowledged that the reflective process they had undertaken helped them to confront their particular practice issues. Some of the practical issues that were addressed included: learning to discern between ideal and real perceptions of midwifery practice; being motivated to do something; generating solutions to problems; looking at themselves and their practices; learning to be assertive; acknowledging that change is difficult; and looking at reasons for frustration and some dynamics of relationships.

Discerning between ideal and real

It's good for that and it also makes you think of what you really are doing . . . about the way you see yourself and the way you actually practise and it's good for bringing yourself back to reality because you have all these ideals for yourself. But it's good to reflect on what you are actually doing, to see if you are actually keeping up with your ideals. Sometimes you fall a bit short of your ideals, but that's because we are human beings as well. It's been really interesting, I found it's been good. (Participant A)

I feel that a lot of midwives could get a lot out of it and just reflecting on their practice and seeing what they actually say they're doing but what they actually are doing. Are they doing what they say they are doing? (Participant C)

Being motivated to do something

If I hadn't been doing this reflective practice at this time, I wouldn't have confronted the woman about this situation and I would have carried it with me, negative thoughts about that person for, probably, forever. It was only through reflection that I realised really that it was an unresolved matter for me and I thought of it several times and each time there was more reflection that went on. It just sort of kept tumbling on and on. That just wouldn't have happened if I hadn't have been doing this reflective practice, at all. So, nothing would have been resolved at all. Instead of having a negative thing to carry around with me now, I have a positive memory.

I think it made me delve more into some problems and find solutions to them, whereas I probably would have found what I thought were solutions, but I think I've got better solutions now. (Participant E)

113

Generating solution to problems

I had an incident involving a really aggressive partner . . . the whole incident was very upsetting for the midwife involved. It was also very stressful for me, because we were confronted with this guy, who was terribly aggressive towards all of the health professionals around him, one girl in particular. That was a situation that I hadn't really come up against . . . So, what we did as part of my reflection on that, we had an inservice grouping and going over of the incident and talking about what had happened, which as part of a reflection of my practice, I thought was very useful. It came out quite effectively actually, because the girl that was involved was able to understand how I'd felt about the whole situation. She had a totally different slant on what she thought I had thought. She had thought that I had thought she wasn't doing her job properly and that she had provoked him and things like that. But, I hadn't thought that at all. In fact, just the opposite, actually. So, for me the reflection was very positive, and for her also. So, I think that if we weren't doing the reflective practice module, well, we probably would have talked about it, but maybe not to the depth that we did. (Participant F)

Looking at self and practices

Just looking at myself and my practices, it has certainly been a learning experience for me. (Participant H)

Learning to be assertive

[I've learned to] just stand up for myself more. I think I've found that. I think, reflecting back on this and looking at my practice, I have actually, these last few months, been standing up for myself more. Before, I'd sort of sometimes just go with the flow. (Participant D)

Yes [the journal helped]. It did help me a lot in that way in that where I was probably becoming a bit blasé in thinking 'Well if they want me to stay here, I'm quite happy to stay here because I'm confident here, but if I went into the Labour Ward situation, I would be a little uncertain for a bit and no one likes that sort of feeling.' So, it took me a while to assert, to want to assert it, to get back to where I was before because no one likes feeling not in control. I think it helped me to realise what was happening and just go for what I wanted again. (Participant D)

Change is difficult

I think [I've learned] . . . people that won't change, refuse to change and that sort of really gets me riled, because we are changing all the time, so that we can introduce more things to help the women that we are looking after and people that won't change really get me going. You try and prod them, but it's hard. That's another thing I find hard, especially when your nursing manager sometimes puts obstacles in front of you as well when you are trying to do the best you can for the ladies and they stay in the dark ages. (Participant G)

Looking at reasons for frustration

I'm finding that it's made me very frustrated in my practice and made me look at why I was frustrated and that sort of hopefully had changed what I was doing in that because I was talking about it. I was talking to people more at work about what was really my big problem. People became more aware and started to help me change it and get it to what is more ideal, well for me, but for everyone else as well. (Participant I)

Other benefits of reflective practice

There was unanimous agreement that the process was useful in particular ways, including for clarifying issues, reviewing practice, looking back at achievements and changes, as an outlet for talking about stresses, and because of the variety of things to discuss.

LEARNING TO VALUE YOURSELF

One of the most difficult lessons you may have to learn in life is to value yourself. In my work I have noticed that nurses and midwives express feelings of low self-esteem and lack of worthiness, and they often seem to spend their time trying to gain acknowledgment from other people such as friends, family members, work peers and superiors. One of the valuable aspects of reflective practice is that you may learn to look at yourself and acknowledge that you are OK, and that you as a person are of value.

These questions are posed for a personal check of how you feel about yourself at this moment:

- Are you at ease with who you are as a person?
- How do you feel about yourself generally?
- On a scale of 1 to 10, the latter being a high, where do you place yourself for feelings of self esteem and worthiness? Why?
- When someone asks you what you do for a living, what do you say?

Learning to value yourself as a nurse or midwife

Over the years I have been working with nurses, the one phrase I have heard repeatedly is: 'I am just a nurse!' I am not sure if midwives say something similar, because I have not worked with them as much. At the basis of a statement such as this is the assumption that, relative to other professions, nursing is insig-nificant in terms of prestige and power. There could also be a sense of familiarity with the work that somehow renders it less important, along the lines of 'If I can do it, anyone can!' Another interesting explanation of the tendency to 'play down' the importance of nursing or midwifery is the lack of value people place in large numbers. There are many nurses and midwives employed within health care systems around the world, playing an integral part in caring for people in need of health care. Because there are so many of them, nurses and midwives may assume that they are less valuable than other 'specialists' who hold relatively rare and better paid health care positions.

Nursing and midwifery is valuable work and, by extension, nurses and midwives are valuable practitioners. When nurses and midwives value their work as practitioners, they value themselves as people who can make important contributions to other people's lives. It is possible that nurses and midwives do not understand the nature and effects of their work, and that part of their struggle to value themselves as practitioners comes from not realising the power they have in their work to make a positive difference to people. Reflective practice enables nurses and midwives to examine their actions at close range and to make sense of their work. By reflecting in and on their practice, they begin to appreciate what they do and how they do it, in terms of its contribution to humanity.

> Do you value yourself as a practitioner? Why?
>   In your journal, record your responses to this reflector so that you can refer to it some time in the future to see if your view on this question is changing due to reflective practice.

Learning to be alert to practice

Through reflective you develop skills in being able to watch yourself in action, during the course of your workday, noticing the nature of interactions and their outcomes. It will be as though you have become a full-time participant observer of your practice activities and situation. This means that work takes on an interesting dimension as though your eyes are cameras catching moments of your work life, keeping a sharper focus on what is happening, to whom, where, when, how and why. Being alert to practice also allows you to replay your experiences at a later time for further reflection on action. Being alert to practice means that you notice more and become clearer about the determinants of given situations, allowing you to make sense of your experiences as a source of learning.

Learning to make work better for yourself

Reflective practice has the potential to improve procedures, interpersonal relationships and organisational factors related to power. Unless you are working in a setting in which all of the procedures are perfect, the relationships are friendly and cooperative, and there are no power plays between people in the organisation, you can make work better for yourself through reflective practice.

Work can be a place where you go simply to earn money, or it can be a place where you earn money and feel relatively happy at the same time. The only way you can change what you have now is to think first, then act. This is what reflective practice is about, because thinking and acting are not simple tasks. If procedures, relationships and power plays are to change positively, systematic and careful reflection is required. The processes described in this book assist you in the kinds of thinking you require and encourage you to take purposeful action to bring about beneficial changes.

Learning to make work better for other people

Reflective practice can work for individuals, and it can work for collectives. All you need to do is work together to intensify the effects of individual efforts. If nurses and midwives collaborated with their peers, there would be so much they could do to improve work conditions and practices. Imagine a group of clinicians working together and sharing their reflective insights. So much could be improved in relation to daily issues, such as procedures, relationships and power plays within the organisation.

It is possible to imagine the organisation thriving through involved employees who are willing to cooperate or contest according to the social and political features of situations. The disciplines of nursing and midwifery would benefit from advances and improvements in practice and build their knowledge through increased reflection, leading to research and publications. While this may seem like a wishful dream to you, it is possible to make work better for yourself and other people. Some evidence that this is the case in nursing and midwifery appears in articles and books (Johns and Freshwater 1998; Street 1995; Taylor et al. 1995) that have documented positive changes which have occurred through reflective practice.

EXCUSES AND REMEDIES

Is a reason the same as an excuse? You may have defended your own behaviour at some time by differentiating 'good' reasons from 'poor' excuses. Reasons seem to have more prestige than excuses, and seem to be founded on something more honourable than mere statements to excuse your behaviour. Therefore, where possible, it is better to offer reasons than excuses, especially when the stakes are high and it is important to win your case for failing to act in anticipated ways. You may think that you have solid reasons for not reflecting. This is a matter for you to decide. In this section I want to expose some of the deterrents to reflection which have been used as reasons or excuses by other would-be reflective practitioners, and suggest ways in which they can remedied.

All too often the reasons for not reflecting outweigh attempts to try to establish reflective practice. There are many excuses for not reflecting and, over many years of teaching, researching and practising reflection, I think I have heard most of them. Most of the excuses come down to five deficiencies that are common to living in general: not enough ability, energy, interest, time and courage. These excuses have been ordered alphabetically, not necessarily in terms of their importance. You might reorder them according to your experience, and you might even add some more, or take some out. Nevertheless, they can be seen as excuses if they fall generally into the category of: 'I know reflection is worthwhile, but . . .'

Not enough ability

'I can't do it' usually means 'I am not smart enough'. Something is radically wrong with this kind of excuse, assuming that this is what is being said and 'not enough ability' is not being put forward as some other excuse. If you are really not smart enough to reflect, it is doubtful that you would be reading this text or thinking about excuses. In other words, the cognitive abilities needed are fundamental to adult life, and they include being able to read, write and think. If you can do all these things, you have the ability for reflection, assuming you are willing to put a little effort into extending your present skills to an analytical level. If you are willing to do this, then you are smart enough.

Not enough energy

This excuse is usually bound up in the constraints of a busy life and not enough energy to go around all your activities and responsibilities. This is reasonable enough when you consider how much nurses and midwives do already in the course of their work lives. Feeling tired and worn out is part and parcel of clinical work, it seems, and you only need look at how hard nurses and midwives work to realise that this excuse is fair enough. However, if life is reliant on energy and there is only a certain amount allotted to each day, the question may become: 'What things matter enough to me to expend some energy on them?' If you can allot enough energy to reflection, you may find that you save time overall through dealing more effectively with work issues and experiencing greater job satisfaction.

Not enough interest

If reflection does not sound interesting to you, it may not be time for you to embark on it just yet, although I am hoping that this book inspires you to become more interested and active. The trouble is, as humans we cannot avoid reflection of some kind and it will probably not be long before you begin to wonder what reflective processes are all about and whether it would be worth investing yourself in them. My argument is this: if you work, you have to think. If you think, it may as well be as effectively as possible. If you want to be as effective as you can at work, you need to reflect systematically on what you think and do and how it might be done differently. This being so, it is about time you worked up some interest in reflective processes at work.

Not enough time

Life is crowded for busy people, especially if they are holding down a job, a family life, and trying to have some fun somewhere in between. I suppose this is the excuse I hear most frequently from nurses and midwives and it is the one I make to myself most often. If you are having trouble finding time to do things, I can empathise! It is such a problem for me, in fact, that I have done a lot of thinking about it and this is what I have resolved to myself. I sometimes hear myself saying: 'I can't find time!' Now, this implies that I have lost it or misplaced it somewhere and that by finding it I will have more time. I've come to realise that time is not waiting to be recovered from some hidden place; rather, it is available to me immediately and all I have to do is to set it aside and plan to use it at the next possible opportunity. I try to think about 'making' time instead of 'finding' it, so I am more proactive in claiming it when I need it for a project of some kind. I am also working on the issue of prioritising my time to ensure that the important tasks I have to do are attended to on time. This does not mean I manage my time issues well, but that I am aware of them and I try to address them. Is it time for you to stop looking for time and simply make it, so that you can become a reflective practitioner?

Not enough courage

Fear is a human condition and courage can desert us at any time. It takes courage to embark on something new and challenging and it is entirely understandable if deep down you have fears related to reflecting on your practice. What are the scary bits about reflecting? Are you afraid of getting started, or of what you might uncover along the way? Are you afraid that when you reflect on issues and locate solutions that you may not have the 'wherewithall' to carry out your plans of action? I have news for you. You are not alone, and more power to you for having the guts to admit to yourself that you lack courage. Daily life presents challenges and success in living depends to some extent on your ability to undertake autonomous action, to propel yourself into each day and to interact within it. I have found that facing some challenges is far less scary than my imagination of them. In other words, when I get in there and take each step at a time, I find I can get through most challenges. This book prepares you for the challenges of reflective practice and all that remains is for you to use the processes, one step at a time, and to move forward at the rate which is most comfortable for you. Take heart and be courageous—bit by bit.

What are your usual excuses for not committing yourself to activities you suspect are helpful for you?

Do you think that any of the previous excuses might apply to you as you begin your journey as a reflective practitioner?

Do you have any ideas on how you might be able to enhance your ability, energy, interest, time and courage for reflective practice?

HOW TO ENHANCE YOUR ABILITY, ENERGY, INTEREST, TIME AND COURAGE

If you think that you do not have enough ability, energy, interest, time and courage, this can be remedied. I have a very interesting rationale for making this claim. I am a self-confessed optimist. I am a product of a Baptist Sunday School beginning and even though I have dropped the rule-ridden religiosity I had as an adolescent, I have retained a sense of spirituality and the goodness of humans as 'sparks of the Divine'. This means that I think people have inbuilt features such as ability, energy, interest, time and courage. It is simply a matter of them recognising themselves as potentially capable of being and doing most things and tapping into all they are or can be. In short, even if you think that you are 'a hopeless case', I don't agree. I offer you some overall strategies for improving the way you view and organise your life and in the process you may collect some extra ability, energy, interest, time and courage and anything else you feel you are lacking.

Life-enabling strategies

An important point to remember is that self-work is always 'work in progress' and you never quite get it all done. Therefore, don't start out searching for perfection, because you won't find it in yourself or anyone else. All the life-enabling strategies you can muster will not refine you to a point at which you are completed as a perfect product of humanity. Life-enabling strategies simply move you on from where you were yesterday.

Our bodies and lives can stay the same, or they can get better or worse, but they never get finished to perfection. I have a suspicion that we think we can attain perfection and that's what we spend most of our time here trying to do. I am 'work in progress'. Sometimes I 'walk my talk', and sometimes I do not.

With all of this in mind, consider some of these enabling strategies to help you find more of what you need to stay interested, active and purposeful in life and work. What I am offering you now are tips which have worked for me at various times in my life. I have read them in books, and heard them from friends, and tried them with varying degrees of attention and success. Let them 'wash over you' as possibilities for helping your progress. The ideas relate to looking more closely at daily routines, such as food, fluids, rest and exercise. I also discuss the usefulness of stress-management techniques such as meditation, visualisation and time management. An important inside-out enabling technique is to think differently and positively about yourself. I share some thoughts and insights I've had on this important area.

What have we got in life if not a succession of days? This is the way life happens, day after day. Life can be a drag and an effort or it can be interesting and energised. I think my life fits the latter category when I pay attention to my daily routines, such as food, fluids, hygiene, rest and exercise. Daily routines are important.

Food and fluid

You know as well I that the food you eat and the fluids you drink affect how you feel and how healthy you become and remain. My adherence varies to the laws of nutrition. Presently, I am eating less saturated fat and drinking more pure water. I know the 'right thing to do' but I don't always do it. I think the biggest insight for me over the years has been to seek balance in my daily routines. I think it is important to realise that food and fluids make a difference to how I feel about myself and the roles I take in my social life. Although I must admit that, overall, I do not manage this part of my life well, I know that when I try harder to balance my intake of nutritious foods and fluids, I feel better and that life flows along easier.

Exercise

The 1990s have been the decade of physical fitness. We have witnessed the ascendancy of joggers, home gym equipment, exercise clubs, aerobics and so on. When it comes to exercise I usually opt for moving my muscles as part of a natural and enjoyable pursuit, such as walking in the bush or on the beach, swimming and gardening. I have respect for people who choose to get sweaty in 'workouts' such as power walking, jogging, and non-competitive and competitive sports. I appreciate that they derive great benefit from the personal challenge and teamwork, while they get fit. You need to discover which kinds of exercise suit you best and how much attention you would like to devote to them. Feeling fitter is related definitely and directly to feeling better.

Rest and relaxation

The 1970s taught us that it is important to relax and many of us are still trying to learn this important lesson. Isn't it strange that, now we know what stress is, we seem to have forgotten how to relax. In trying to get a balance of rest and exercise, I know I need to be more interested in exercise as I have no trouble at all with finding rest and relaxation. Find a hobby you enjoy and do it for fun and relaxation, not for competitive purposes or as source of income if you can avoid it, because when a hobby becomes a necessity it can lose a lot of its charm and usefulness as a means of relaxation.

Meditation

My stress management consists of meditation, visualisation and time management and I have come to understand them in my own way. I simply share a few of these ideas with you. I learned to meditate in 1974 when I was 23 years of age. This was the single most important gift that I could ever have given myself. It was around the time that Maharishi Yogi and the Beatles made meditation respectable to Westerners as a stress-management technique. My regular practice of meditation was such a life-altering event that my mother remarked one day that I had become a lot 'nicer'. Although this was a rather 'backhanded' compliment, I took it well and went on to become a more centred and stable person because of meditation.

If you do not know how to meditate, visit a 'new age' book shop and you will find many resources on the subject, such as books, tapes, compact discs and offers of training in techniques. You can experience meditation by this simple technique. Take the phone off the hook, find a quiet place, sit in a chair with your back straight, put your feet flat on the floor, rest your hands in your lap, shut your eyes, rest quietly until you settle, let your body relax, then think slowly and softly on the sound: 'OM'. Repeat it gently to yourself, either silently within or out loud. Don't work hard at it, just let the sound move in and out with your breath. Do this for 20 minutes or until you feel it has finished. If you can meditate twice a day for 20 minutes with this or another technique you discover, that would be good, but if you can't, do it when you can. You may notice that your pulse rate and blood pressure decrease and that you feel calmer generally. Altogether, meditation can become an important life-enabling strategy for you.

Guided visualisation

In a guided visualisation you 'see' a positive scene which gives you a sense of deep relaxation. These scenes are described on audiotape and you prepare yourself in a way similar to meditation and listen to the narrator guide you through the experience. The scene may be of a walk through a rainforest or along a beach, noticing the colours and textures of the natural surroundings. Some people can see the colours and all of the features of the scene as it is described, while other people experience a sense of peace and calm with no or few visual cues. Usually the tape contains messages, which are always positive, telling you that you are safe, protected, loved and secure, as you experience deep relaxation. Visualisation tapes can be purchased from 'new age' stores, and you need to listen for a while to choose one which will suit your needs. This is a good stress-management technique when you think you may have some difficulty getting 'into' a meditation, because you simply turn on a tape and are guided through the experience.

Time management

For me, time management is about planning to make time for everything in my life. I use a diary to keep me aware of what is due, when and where. I consult my diary often to ensure that I am keeping up with my promises to attend this, speak here, write that and so on. When I have a big event coming up, such as a conference presentation, I write notes to myself in the diary well ahead of time, to ensure that I have enough time to prepare sufficiently. I also use daily checklists to prioritise the important tasks, which must be done before a certain time limit, especially if I have many jobs competing for my attention. Listing jobs on paper takes away the anxiety of trying to remember them. When I pre-plan, I ask for help if I need it, and I delegate as appropriate to other available and willing people. One of my biggest life lessons to date has been learning that I do not have to do everything myself and that other people are as capable as I am of doing a good job. Actually, I've learned that lesson so well that I would gladly accept more help if I could find it! If you learn how to organise your time more effectively, you may find that your life is enhanced greatly when you make more time for important people and events.

Thinking differently and positively

It was a major revelation to me when I realised that I could take the biggest part in determining my moods, emotions, thoughts, actions and relationships. I had heard this interesting concept before—that I was in charge of my life—but it took some time for the message to sink in. What a difference it made when I started taking responsibility for myself! I realised that I could experience my moods, emotions and thoughts, but they did not have to take me over and wreck my day entirely. After a time of languishing in a delectable emotion such as self-pity, blame, guilt, fear and so on, I could actually move on and get over it! I also realised that I did not have to think negatively about myself or anything or anybody else. This was an interesting one, because it meant I would have to find someone else to blame if things went wrong, or maybe blame was a transitory and unhelpful emotion anyway.

Having worked through my ownership of my moods, emotions and thoughts, I realised that it had positive flow-on effects for my actions and relationships. I could choose to act autonomously according to my well-considered opinions and judgments, or hunches and intuitions, and to experience a wide variety of options, choices and life experiences. For example,

I could decide about relationships with people with whom I wanted to spend time.

I find it amusing that some of my biggest insights and life changes come from the simplest messages, such as 'think differently and positively about yourself'. Related to this idea is one of life's great puzzles—that people spend most of their lives searching for love and learning how to love themselves. As I grow older, I realise that the two are connected. It seems to me that I looked outside myself for love because I had not learned to love myself. I thought I could find love somewhere else and that it relied on the cooperation and approval of other people, such as my family, friends and associates. The reason I share these observations is to make the point that I learned to love, accept, acknowledge myself and give myself permission to think positively about myself and so can you.

At the beginning of this section on life-enabling strategies, I owned up to my optimistic views about humanity and why I hold these views. What is your basic view of humanity? How does this view influence you in the ways you practise?

Do you have any other life-enabling strategies which differ from mine? What are they? Why do they work for you?

Possibilities for future reflective practice

In the research project I have mentioned throughout this chapter (Taylor et al. 1995), participants talked about their hopes for continuing reflective practice with colleagues and for themselves. This was explored in relation to the potential of the process for creating open discussion of midwifery practice, the usefulness of the approach as a general model of problem solving and in terms of personal commitments to continuing reflection. I have included the following comments from clinicians to show you that there is value in reflective practice and that it worth any time and effort you can give to it.

Encouraging open discussion of practice

> Well, I really think it's a good idea to encourage others to reflect on their practice. Like at work, we do tend to talk a lot about what we're doing. I tend to talk more to the girls that are into the same sort of things that I'm into and we sort of encourage each other in what we want to achieve. (Participant B)

A general model of problem solving

Virginia [a co-researcher] reported:

> He [a participant] is using reflection across his life. On the farm [at home] he sets goals, and if a problem occurs he does not get angry but thinks about solutions. He passed on information about reflection to one midwife he worked with who was impressed by it. He believes it is relationships at work which push his buttons. He feels he does things differently now because of reflection.

Continuing reflection

> I think I'll continue writing in (the log), about various incidents. (Participant I)
>
> Well I made a deal with myself that I would continue until the end of the year and I have talked to someone to be a critical friend. I thought that by another six months, it would come without having to make a concerted effort to do it. Yes, it works. (Participant J)

SUMMARY

In this chapter, I reviewed some literature on professions and professionals and discussed why reflection is valuable for all practitioners, especially nurses and midwives. I emphasised the value of being a reflective practitioner and learning to value yourself as a person and as a nurse or midwife. I explained that part of this process is about learning to be alert to your practice, to make things better for yourself, other people, the organisation in which you work, and for your practice discipline. I concluded this chapter by looking at some excuses used often to avoid reflective practice and some strategies for thinking differently and positively about yourself as you become a reflective practitioner.

6

Types of reflection

Reflection can be used for many purposes, depending on how and when it is done, by whom and why. Reflection happens irrespective of the time of day, or whether you are at work or home, and the reflective insights gained may have applications for any sphere of your life.

In this chapter, after sounding a note of caution about the use of categories, I will introduce three main types of reflection nurses and midwives can use in their work and adapt to their personal lives if they wish. As the basis for understanding how knowledge is related to reflection, I then introduce some nursing and midwifery authors who have categorised ways of knowing. After that I will describe empirical, interpretive and critical knowledge and Habermas's 'knowledge-constitutive interests' so that you can see how they relate to the kinds of reflection highlighted in this book. Finally I introduce technical, practical and emancipatory reflection and highlight their relative merits, so that you can decide which type or combination of types of reflection to use for your practice issues.

CAUTION ABOUT CATEGORIES

I tend to get nervous at the prospect of putting ideas in neat, fixed categories, because the older I become, the more I realise that concepts do not necessarily fit in certain boxes with the lid firmly on. This is because I realise more and more how everything is connected understand that and as soon as I attempt to compile or classify according to a defined type or category, something pops up which does not quite fit.

If you have read about postmodern thinking, you may have found that this approach resists putting knowledge forms into discrete categories, because of reservations about how prescriptive these 'grand narratives' become in the way people begin to see themselves, the world around them and the way knowledge is constructed within it. While I may have my own reservations about categorising knowledge and while I may realise that more caution is expressed by other people (Baudrillard 1988; Giroux 1990), I still realise how difficult it is for students of any new ideas to start off without structure and content which can be shifted into categories as though it had some 'concrete' form. An amorphous, postmodern, no-boundaries approach to understanding may come with increased knowledge over time, but it is my experience as a teacher and learner over many years that understanding does not appear in this way to a novice. This is why I am suggesting in this chapter that it is possible to imagine three types of reflection, which have distinct features according to the kind of knowledge they generate.

Elsewhere (Taylor in Johns and Freshwater 1998: 134–50) I have written about three broad categories of nursing and midwifery knowledge: empirical, interpretive and critical. Some of this information will be reiterated briefly in this chapter, to show the connections between ways of knowing and reflecting. In effect, I will be suggesting that empirical knowledge comes from technical reflection, interpretive knowledge comes from practical reflection, and critical knowledge comes from emancipatory reflection. This is not saying anything novel, as these categories have been written about previously in relation to education (Mezirow 1981) and research (Carr and Kemmis 1984). That these categories have been used successfully elsewhere suggests that they are useful, even though there are cautionary notes to be heeded about trying to fit ideas into categories.

It is important to consider these categories as ways of creating a tidy framework on which to hang certain broad principles. The tendency to create a structure fits the assumption that there are major paradigms, or world views of knowledge, which can accommodate large chunks of related ideas. It would be short-sighted to have an absolute conviction that there are only three forms of knowledge and reflection. I do not intend that you should think like this. The categories I am suggesting are ways of structuring your thinking until you have the confidence you need to take the conceptual boxes away so that you can roam freely in open fields of unclassified knowledge and reflection.

It is also important that you do not think that these three forms of knowledge and reflection are opposed to one another or mutually exclusive, because they actually share common features and at times they can merge into one another. All three approaches can use similar ways of thinking, even though in some cases it seems a fairly 'clean cut' decision as to the specific type of thinking to use in particular instances. For example, the tasks involved in technical reflection would most probably be best served by a high degree of rationality of a 'scientific model' kind. In relation to these categories not being mutually exclusive, it may transpire, for instance, that emancipatory reflection might include some aspects of scientific rationality—say, for example, if part of the process involves changing outmoded clinical procedures to something which can be shown to demonstrate better practice.

So you can see that the categories I suggest in this book may be useful for you to get a firm hold on reflection, but they are not meant to be absolute, indisputable, inflexible systems that lock you in. Neither are they opposed to one another or mutually exclusive. In the future, when you become more adept at being a reflective practitioner, you may realise that you are doing reflection which leans towards a specific type, but which does not necessarily exclude other possibilities.

Thinking about knowledge categories

What types of knowledge do you use at work? Be as creative as you can and use any words you like to write a list. Don't worry if the types overlap or do not agree with any categories described in this book. Look at your list of categories and ask yourself: 'Do these types of knowledge represent everything I know or need to know about my work?' If you think that you have a complete list of categories, try to think of exceptions to the rule, in which these categories do not apply.

Do you think that any list of knowledge categories explains all you know or need to know in your work? Why? Write some notes in your journal about these questions and refer to them whenever you are puzzling about issues concerning with knowledge.

KNOWLEDGE IN NURSING AND MIDWIFERY

The history of knowledge has been traced though the study of many different disciplines, structured under the broad classifications of the humanities and sciences. Within each of these main branches of knowledge are two implicit concerns of human knowledge and existence, which are explored through epistemology and ontology. *Epistemology* concerns itself with knowledge generation and validation, meaning that it tries to ascertain how to make new knowledge and how to judge whether it is trustworthy and 'true'. *Ontology* is the meaning of the human existence. These two main foci of human interest are related to one another if you accept the argument that knowing about human existence is the basis for knowing the answers to any questions humans might pose (Heidegger 1962; Gadamer 1975).

There are many ways of thinking about knowledge and existence. In nursing and midwifery, several approaches have been suggested (Allen et al. 1986; Carper 1978; Chinn and Kramer 1991; Parse 1987). Carper (1978) suggests four fundamental patterns of knowing in nursing: empirics, the science of nursing; esthetics, the art of nursing; the component of personal knowledge in nursing; and ethics, the moral component.

Chinn and Kramer (1991: 15) support Carper but warn nurses and midwives that if these categories are removed from the context of the whole of knowing, they could lead to 'patterns gone wild'. Each form has the potential for unbalanced applications—for example, empirics can result in control and manipulation; ethics can produce rigid doctrine and insensitivity to the rights of others; personal knowing can produce isolation and self-distortion; and esthetics has the potential for producing prejudice, bigotry and lack of appreciation for meaning.

Allen et al. (1986: 23) describe three paradigms for generating knowledge within nursing and midwifery: the empirico-analytical paradigm, Heideggerian phenomenology and critical social theory. These paradigms align with Habermas's technical, practical and emancipatory categorisations of 'knowledge-constitutive interests' respectively.

Parse (1987) categorises her own work into the Simultaneity paradigm and claims that it is a human science approach to nursing, which views a person as a unitary being in continuous mutual interrelationship with the environment. This paradigm aligns knowledge with the concept of holism and the interconnectedness of people and their environment.

Using the information in the section above, draw a model which represents knowledge in nursing and midwifery. This means that you will try to include all of the authors' ideas and indicate connections between them.

You might like to compare this model with the list you prepared previously of the categories of knowledge you use at work. How are they similar and different? You might like to amend your list in light of new information represented in the model of knowledge in nursing and midwifery.

Although each of these approaches has merit, the approach taken in this book will be to use the categories suggested by Habermas (1972) of empirical, interpretive and critical paradigms of knowledge. As you read further in this chapter, you will notice that these three forms are able to explain human knowledge as cognitive interests, aspects of social existence, reflection and foci of learning. At this stage, however, I will describe empirical, interpretive and critical knowledge so that you can see how they relate to the kinds of reflection highlighted in this book.

Empirical knowledge

Empirical knowledge is generated and tested through 'the scientific method'. The scientific method is a set of rules for gaining knowledge through a systematic and rigorous procedure. Scientific inquiry ensures that knowledge can be tested over and over again and found to be accurate and consistent (reliability). It also ensures that it tests what it actually intends (validity) rather than other factors that are there extra or unnoticed (extraneous variables). To achieve this, scientific knowledge is rendered as free as possible from the distorting influences of people, such as their prejudices, intentions and emotions (subjectivity). In other words, empirical knowledge needs to show that due consideration has been given to achieving objectivity.

Another requirement of empirical knowledge is that the only research questions that can be asked legitimately are those which can be structured in ways that can be observed and analysed (by empirico-analytical means) and measured by numbers, percentages and statistics (quantified). This is why research using the scientific method is also referred to as empirico-analytical and/or quantitative research. The scientific method reduces areas of inquiry to their smallest parts (reductionism) in order to study them. This idea assumes that all empirical knowledge is waiting to be discovered and assembled, as absolute knowledge. The reason empirical knowledge is reductionist is that it attempts to find cause and effect links between certain objects and subjects (variables), which are controlled and manipulated carefully. Empirical knowledge confirms or disputes the degree of certainty in cause and effect relationships, by demonstrating significance statistically. This allows empirical knowledge to claim to be predictive and generalisable with some confidence that the conclusions are truthful, real and trustworthy, and not just happening by chance. The outcomes are achieved mainly through rational deductive thinking processes which move systematically from broad to focused inferences.

In summary, the features of the scientific method generate and validate empirical knowledge through rigorous means such as reliability, validity, and control and manipulation of variables, to produce objective data that can be quantified to demonstrate the degree of statistical significance in cause and effect relationships. The outcomes of this method for the generation of empirical knowledge include description of what is, prediction for what might be, and change through new knowledge discoveries. The success of empirical knowledge is evident in nursing and midwifery through the constant evolution of newer and safer technical nursing and midwifery procedures.

Identifying empirical knowledge

List four clinical procedures you use in your work.

Why is it important for these procedures to be described and performed objectively?

How do you decide that these procedures are trustworthy?

At what point would you decide that these procedures were no longer trustworthy?

Interpretive knowledge

People are central to interpretive knowledge, because of their perceptions of their life experiences and their ability to communicate them. The underlying concepts of interpretive knowledge include interpersonal understanding through attention to lived experience, context and subjectivity. There is so much to say about each of these concepts, but I will try to make them as succinct as possible, so that you have a clear idea of their essential features.

Lived experience means knowing what it is like to live a life in a particular time, place and set of circumstances. Humans have the potential for reflecting on lived experiences. Other living beings such as animals may also have lived experiences, but they are relatively unable to communicate them, therefore lived experience is described in terms of human existence only. A philosopher named Dilthey (1985) suggests that lived experience is awareness of life without thinking about it, a pre-reflexive consciousness of life. He explains (1985: 223) that:

[a] lived experience does not confront me as something perceived or represented; it is not given to me, but the reality of the lived experience is there-for-me because I have reflexive awareness of it, because I possess it immediately as belonging to me in some sense. Only in thought does it become objective.

From this description, you can see that Dilthey thinks that lived experience happens before reflection, like a grasp of events not requiring objective thought. It is only through reflection, however, that sense is made of lived experience.

In agreement with Dilthey's (1985) understanding of lived experience, Dreyfus (1979, in Benner and Wrubel 1989: 83) claims that 'we are able to move around in the everyday world because our understanding is always situated and our actions are typically only as orderly as the situation demands'. Novel situations may be managed with reference to like situations of which people have had previous experience. This seems true of nursing and midwifery practice. Practitioners are very familiar with the work setting and circumstances, and thus they feel ready for what may transpire as part of the work day. Nurses and midwives have a knack of knowing what to do and how to do it in certain unforeseen circumstances. One explanation for this is their lived experience of being a practitioner.

Context means all of the features of the time and place in which people find themselves, in which they locate their lives. People live their daily lives in the moment, yet they also remain connected to their past and future (Heidegger 1962). People cannot help but be placed, and involved in, a particular time and place, which gives a sense of familiarity. Context provides relative security for daily activity, because so many things can happen in an ever-changing world. Nurses and midwives work out what to do and how to do it in any situation by making personal applications to their own life issues, worries and stories, and to their sense of time, habits and favoured rituals and patterns of behaviour in various groups. They also pay attention to how they feel and what sense they make of it based on experience.

Subjectivity refers to the individual's sensing of inner and external events, which does not make a universal claim to be true for everyone and for all things at all times and in all places. Subjectivity includes personal experiences and truths, that may or may not be like other people's subjective experiences and

137

truths. 'Intersubjectivity' refers to how individuals take account of one another in the social world to make sense of their experiences. Nursing and midwifery occur in social contexts in which intersubjective meanings are generated, because clinicians interpret their work experiences from their respective person-to-person viewpoints.

In summary, interpretive knowledge emerges from the perspectives of people engaged actively in their lives and it includes and values what people feel and think. Judgments as to the usefulness and 'truthfulness' of the accounts are based on the relative indicators, such as the nature of lived experience, context and subjectivity.

Identifying interpretive knowledge

Whenever you assign personal meaning to events and interpersonal relationships in your life, you are using interpretive knowledge.

Think of an interpersonal encounter you have had today. It could be as simple as greeting a friend as you pass, or it could be as complex as a heated argument with someone.

To understand how you use interpretive knowledge, keep today's encounter in mind and respond to these questions in your journal:

- What were the contextual features of the encounter? In other words, where, when, how and with whom did this encounter happen?
- What were the subjective features of the encounter—that is, what did you think and feel about the encounter?
- What were the intersubjective features of the encounter—how did you interpret the encounter compared with other similar interpersonal meetings?

The statements you have written in response to this reflector represent interpretations of a situation. As you can see, interpretive knowledge plays a large part in daily life as humans make sense of their existence.

Critical knowledge

Critical knowledge is derived from some key ideas in critical social science, which emerged from the social and epistemological needs that presented after World War I. In a nutshell, a group of philosophers of the Frankfurt School decided that a way of generating knowledge other than through the scientific method was needed to open up new thinking about human knowing and experience, in order to prevent future wars and domination by oppressive regimes. Critical knowledge has the potential to be emancipatory—that is, it can free people from the oppression of their entrenched social and personal conditions.

The need for emancipation comes from the assumption that certain people, in the circumstances in which they find them selves, may suffer oppression and constraints of some kind at the hands of other people and regimes. Freedom from oppression comes from being aware that it is happening in terms of historical, social, political, cultural and economic determinants and from finding the means to do something about it. Critical knowledge and theorising seek to look into what is promoted as the status quo of various repressive social contexts, to discover and expose the forces that maintain them for their particular advantages. This means that they look at the way life is and ask how it might be different and better for the majority of people, not just for the privileged few.

Critical knowledge includes consideration of lived experience, context and intersubjectivity; other related key ideas are false consciousness, hegemony, reification, emancipation and empowerment. I will explain each of these latter terms briefly. You will see that the first three words describe the oppressive potential of social life, and the last two words provide some optimism about how repressive circumstances can be overcome.

False consciousness is the 'systematic ignorance that the members of . . . society have about themselves and their society' (Fay 1987: 27). Critical knowledge attempts to critique firmly held individual and collective ignorance to change this self-defeating consciousness and transform society itself. Nurses and midwives might relate to this concept as practitioners working in bureaucratic settings where oppressive daily rituals remain unquestioned because they are unnoticed. For example, underlying assumptions as to why nurses and midwives continue to accept power structures in their workplace may not be examined.

Hegemony means the ascendancy or domination of one power over another. In a critical social science interpretation, it refers to the ways in which some social systems, and the people in them, give the impression that they are unassailable, and that the conditions they have produced are not only good, but also appropriate for the people over whom they have control. In nursing and midwifery, this might mean that nurses come to think that the hospital bureaucracy is not only necessary, but also conducive to their welfare, and that the oppressive elements within it, such as dominating relationships and difficult work conditions, cannot and should not be changed. Thus hegemony would have nurses and midwives believe that they can do little to change their work lives.

Fay (1987: 92) explains that *reification* means 'making into a thing'. He defines it as 'taking what are essential activities and treating them as if they operated according to a given set of laws independently of the wishes of the social actors who engage in them'. These laws of social life are assigned a power of their own. For example, a female nurse or midwife may assume that, as a woman, it is a given that she will be subordinate to doctors who are often males, so she acts in accordance with that assumption and fetches, carries, cleans up and generally accedes to the doctor's orders.

Emancipation means freedom, and it infers that one is free from something and free towards something. Critical knowledge claims to be helpful in emancipating people from their present conditions to something better. Emancipation for nurses and midwives, therefore, can mean that they experience freedom from their own and other people's expectations and roles, and be free to adopt other self-aware and socially aware practices.

Empowerment is the process of giving and accepting power. Critical knowledge is geared towards helping people to find their own power, to liberate them from their oppressive circumstances and self-understandings in those circumstances. Empowerment for nurses and midwives may come about when they have worked through a radical critique of their personal and professional roles and conditions and they have liberated themselves to other possibilities, such as being the patients' advocate and demonstrating and asserting their worth in the health team.

In summary, critical knowledge is potentially liberating for individuals and groups of people, when they realise that they may be living under systematically developed and held misunderstandings about themselves and their social situations. As people and practitioners, nurses and midwives are subject to oppressive social structures, which can be transformed through critical analysis and action.

Identifying critical knowledge

There are many riddles to puzzle over in thinking about critical knowledge.
For example, ask yourself these questions:

- If false consciousness is 'systematic ignorance', how do I know when I have it? In other words, if I am ignorant, I am ignorant, therefore, I do not even know that I am ignorant.
- Also, if I am to be relieved of my ignorance, who decides to do that, and how will they help me?
- How do I know that their awareness is better than mine?
- What influences or forces have made me ignorant?
- What influences or forces can liberate me from my ignorance?

Hegemony and reification are other conceptual puzzles. Using the above questions as guides, write some questions of your own that highlight the puzzles in hegemony and reification. To do this, you will need to review the definitions and treat them as problematic.

In raising these questions about some concepts of critical knowledge, you have actually used a process which questions some claims about the nature of human life. This type of questioning of accepted 'truths' lies at the heart of critical knowledge.

KNOWLEDGE AND HUMAN INTERESTS

Jurgen Habermas, a prominent philosopher and sociologist, expounded a compelling critical theory of knowledge and human interests. I will describe some of these ideas to you now, as they are central to how I decided to set out this book into three kinds of reflection. My description of Habermas's ideas is derived from some of his work (Habermas 1972) and from other writers who have supported his work (Fay 1987; Mezirow 1981).

As a critical theorist, Habermas argued that human knowledge could be categorised as technical, practical and emancipatory, based on primary cognitive interests. He suggested that these areas are 'knowledge-constitutive interests' because they determine categories humans interpret as knowledge. He based this on his reasoning that human experience had been constructed socially by humans, and knowledge and social existence represented identifiable human interests. In other words, he claimed that accumulating and checking on the truthfulness of knowledge, as well as being part of a social structure, really mattered to humans who made these two areas important foci in their lives, to the extent that they were obvious interests. He argued that these interests were based on aspects of social existence, such as work, interaction and power. He connected technical interests to work, practical interests to interaction, and emancipatory interests to power.

Technical interest and work

In Habermas's view, technical interest in work creates 'instrumental action' through which people control and manipulate their environments. This means that people act in accordance with technical rules to generate empirical knowledge. I explained empirical knowledge previously in this chapter, but you may recall that it relates to finding information which can be proven to be correct or incorrect according to the rules of the scientific method. The empirical–analytical sciences have been developed to assist in understanding technical interests relating to work. These sciences are identified readily by their use of quantitative research methods which allow them to generalise results and predict future tendencies for similar effects and outcomes to occur. For nurses and midwives, this means that technical interest is associated with task-related competence, such as clinical procedures. There is an increasing call in nursing and midwifery for evidence as a basis for better practice and many of the work practices that need to be improved require technical interest using objective and systematic lines of inquiry.

Practical interests and interaction

Practical interest involves human interaction, or 'communicative action', which involves reciprocal expectations about behaviour which are defined and understood by the people involved. Social norms, or sets of expectations for behaviour, are created over time by people who are in consensus as to what is expected in certain situations. The social norms are enforced through sanctions, which ensure that people recognise and honour their responsibilities in reciprocal behaviour. If this sounds a bit 'heavy', in a nursing or midwifery context communicative action translates to something as familiar as the communication patterns that are set up by practitioners and the people with whom they come into contact. For example, the ways in which you communicate may differ between people—for example, you may communicate in a certain way with patients' relatives in a waiting room and in a different way with doctors at the unit desk.

Practical interest in communicative action requires ways of understanding it according to the people involved. Its main intentions are to describe and explain human interaction, so this kind of interest is situated in the 'historical–hermeneutic sciences', which are concerned with interpretation and explanation. Some examples of these sciences are history, aesethics and literary studies. Practical understanding is mediated through language which describes and explains the area of interest. Previously I referred to this kind of knowledge as interpretive knowledge, because it intends to understand human interaction through understanding the meaning of experience.

Emancipatory interest and power

Emancipatory interest is rooted in power and creates 'transformative action'. Emancipatory interest involves the interpretive elements as described previously in practical interests, especially as people interpret themselves in terms of their roles and social obligations. However, its main intentions are motivated by 'transformative action' which seeks to provide emancipation from forces which limit people's rational control of their lives. These forces are so influential and taken for granted that they give people the strong impression that they are beyond their control.

The modes of inquiry for exploring and critiquing emancipatory interests associated with power are the critical social sciences. Some examples of critical social sciences include critical forms of sociology, politics and feminism. Critical theorists suggest that people must become conscious 'of how an ideology reflects and distorts moral, social and political reality and what material and psychological factors influence and sustain the false consciousness which it represents—especially reified powers of domination' (Mezirow 1981: 145). The kind of radical critique suggested by Mezirow is necessary for nurses and midwives as they examine the effects of power in their work settings and how situations become entrenched and taken for granted and continue to constrain work relationships and practices.

In summary, in this book I have chosen to refer to three types of reflection, which are derived from Habermas' technical, practical and emancipatory 'knowledge-constitutive interests'. This is not a revolutionary thing to do, as similar approaches have been taken in education and research. Habermas connected technical interests to work, practical interests to interaction, and emancipatory interests to power. Technical interest in work creates 'instrumental action' through which people control and manipulate their environments. Practical interest creates human interaction or 'communicative action', which involves reciprocal expectations about behaviour, defined and understood by the people involved. Emancipatory interest is rooted in power and it creates 'transformative action' through which people can free themselves from forces which limit their rational control of their lives. These interests form the basis of the types of reflection presented in this book. In the next section, I will connect Habermas's 'knowledge-constitutive interests' to technical, practical and emancipatory reflection.

Table 6.1 may help you to distinguish the features of each paradigm according to the cognitive interests related to the kind of reflection, the aspects of social existence, and the action and learning involved.

Table 6.1   Three paradigms of knowledge with associated
cognitive interests, aspects of social existence,
action and learning involved

Paradigm of knowledge	Empirical	Interpretive	Critical
Cognitive interests related to the kind of reflection	Technical	Practical	Emancipatory
Aspect of social existence	Work	Interaction	Power
Action involved	Instrumental	Communicative	Transformative
Learning involved	Task-related competence	Interpersonal	Transformation

THREE TYPES OF REFLECTION

Nurses and midwives engaged in daily practice have the advantage of living their practice, in that they have opportunities to look at their practice to learn from it. When nurses and midwives reflect on what they do, they can make sense of their practice, and imagine and/or bring about changes (Street 1990, 1991; Cox et al. 1991; Taylor et al. 1995). The kinds of changes they desire might direct the kind of reflection they use.

In this section I will highlight the advantages and limitations of technical, practical and emancipatory reflection. I will also suggest that each type is as important as the others and that a type or combination of types may be used according to the requirements of the clinical situation. Because each of these ways of reflecting is important, I have devoted a chapter to each of them in this book. All I am intending to do in this section is to give you a brief introduction to the individual features of technical, practical and emancipatory reflection.

Technical reflection

The scientific model's influence on empirical knowledge is apparent in daily practice. Many innovations and evidence-based adaptations in nursing and midwifery have been possible because of empirical knowledge, which is gained through empirical research and what I am terming technical reflection.

The scientific method and rational, deductive thinking and

145

reflection will allow you to generate and validate empirical knowledge through rigorous means, so that you can be assured that work procedures are based on scientific reasoning. If clinical questions and issues are complex, as they tend to be when they are related to competency in practice, technical reflection may accompany empirical research projects which are based on reliability, validity, and control and manipulation of variables. The technical reflection thus instigated will produce objective data that can be quantified to demonstrate the degree of statistical significance in cause and effect relationships. Technical reflection will allow you to adapt present procedures to make them into better ones. You may also be able to predict likely outcomes for similar procedures.

Technical reflection will help you to improve your instrumental action through technical control and manipulation in devising and improving procedural approaches to your work.

> Make a list of all your work situations and procedures that could benefit from technical reflection. Keep your list until you read more in this book about how to undertake technical reflection, at which point you can work in depth using this process.

Although technical reflection offers a great deal of important knowledge in relation to determining the competency of work practices and procedures, by itself it will not be sufficient to interpret the meaning of what it is like to exist and work in settings that are full of other people who rely on making sense of their interpersonal communication patterns and behaviours.

Technical reflection by itself will not assist you in understanding the social interactions and consensual norms that govern the communication of the people undertaking and receiving the procedures, because it does not have an interest in human interaction and communicative action. Also, technical reflection by itself will not raise your awareness of power relationships between the givers and receivers of procedures and it will not provide a radical critique of the unexamined assumptions about social, economic, historical and cultural influences that underlie the instrumental action in procedural activities, because it does not have an interest in power and transformative action.

Technical reflection methods and processes are explained in detail in Chapter 7.

Practical reflection

Interpretation for description and explanation are the key outcomes of practical reflection, which focuses on human interaction in social existence. Communicative action in nursing or midwifery relates to shared communication of norms and expectations.

Practical reflection offers a means of making sense of human interaction. Through the medium of language, practical reflection will help you to understand the interpersonal basis of human experiences and it will offer you the potential for creating knowledge which interprets the meaning of lived experience, context and subjectivity. It will also offer you the potential for change, based on your raised awareness of the nature of a wide range of communicative matters pertaining to nursing and midwifery.

Make a list of all your work situations and procedures that could benefit from practical reflection. Keep your list until you read more in this book about how to undertake practical reflection, at which point you can work in depth using this process.

However, practical reflection will not offer you the objective means to observe and analyse work procedures through a scientific method, because it does not have an interest in instrumental action. Also, practical reflection will not offer you a radical critique of the constraining forces and power influences within nurses' and midwives' work settings. The reason for this is that, although practical reflection can raise awareness through insights into communicative action, it does not have transformative action as its primary concern.

Practical reflection methods and processes are explained in detail in Chapter 8.

Emancipatory reflection

Emancipatory reflection involves human interaction, but its focus is how people interpret themselves in terms of their roles and social obligations. Emancipatory reflection leads to 'transformative action' which seeks to free nurses and midwives from taken-for-granted assumptions and oppressive forces which limit them and their practice.

Emancipatory reflection provides you with a systematic means of critiquing the power relationships in your workplace and it offers you raised awareness and a new sense of informed consciousness to bring about positive social and political change. Emancipatory reflection also offers nurses and midwives the potential to identify their own misguided and firmly held perceptions of themselves and their roles, to bring about change for the better. The process of emancipatory reflection for change is praxis. Praxis in nursing and midwifery offers clinicians the means for change through collaborative processes that analyse and challenge existing forces and distortions brought about by dominating effects of power in human interaction.

> Make a list of all your work situations and procedures that could benefit from emancipatory reflection. Keep your list until you read more in this book about how to undertake emancipatory reflection, at which point you can work in depth using this process.

Even though emancipatory reflection will provide a critique of power in your work setting and relationships, it will not offer you a central focus on the technical interest of procedures at work, because it does not have an abiding and primary interest in instrumental action. Also, even though it begins with analyses of social interactions and consensual norms that govern human communication, emancipatory reflection is more concerned with examining the distortions that occur in communicative action than it is in generating a rich description of the meaning of human experience as it is lived by people involved in the practice of nursing and midwifery.

Emancipatory reflection methods and processes are explained in detail in Chapter 9.

CHOOSING A TYPE OF REFLECTION

There is no form of reflection which is better than another; each has its own value for different purposes. This is the same as saying that no one form of knowledge is superior to another. For a long time, nurses and midwives thought they had to imitate the medical model and the scientific method in the way they thought about and researched their work. As a consequence of scientific approaches, a culture developed which included traditions such as objective language in conversations and nurses' and midwives' notes, and reductionist tendencies to treat people as diagnoses requiring specific attention to the affected body part. Added to this was a strong belief that the only kind of research that was useful and valid was quantitative, because it involved prediction, control, numbers and statistics, which were seen to serve medical practice well, and could thus benefit nursing and midwifery. Some nurses and midwives may have moved on somewhat from the days of medical domination and scientific rationality, but many of them may not be aware of the choices they can make in making sense of their practice.

All kinds of knowledge can be generated through reflection, and nurses and midwives can benefit from a range of reflective processes. The first set of questions you should ask yourself in choosing a specific type or combination of types of reflection consists of: 'What do I want to know through reflection?' 'Why do I want to know it?' 'What questions will stimulate and guide my reflections and lead me to the answers I am seeking?' 'Is my primary focus on work procedures, human interaction or power relationships, or a combination of these interests?'

In the section above I have described the features of technical, practical and emancipatory reflection. I think that finding a balance for using types of knowledge and reflection is important, because knowledge exists for all sorts of purposes and the reflective means nurses and midwives use will depend on what they need to achieve. Getting back to a point I made previously, the categories of reflection are artificial—they do not exist in isolation from one another and they are not mutually exclusive. Remember this as you read on through this book, so that your choices can be informed by broader considerations than choosing one type of reflection over another. If you can develop a reflective consciousness based on balance and context, it will serve you well in deciding how to reflect on any issues which present themselves in your practice.

SUMMARY

In this chapter, I cautioned you about the use of categories and introduced three main types of reflection you can use in your work and adapt to your life if you wish. As the basis for understanding how knowledge is related to reflection, I introduced some nursing and midwifery authors who have categorised ways of knowing. After that I described empirical, interpretive and critical knowledge and Habermas's 'knowledge-constitutive interests' so that you could see how they relate to the kinds of reflection highlighted in this book. Finally I introduced technical, practical and emancipatory reflection and highlighted their relative merits, so that you can decide on which type or combination of types of reflection to use for your practice issues.

7

Technical reflection

- Are you undertaking clinical procedures which you suspect may be of minimal or no value?
- How long is it since someone raised the issue that work practices may be outdated and even counter-productive?
- Are your hospital policies out of touch with clinical realities?
- Do you ever get the feeling that certain nursing or midwifery procedures could be done better or that some of them should be 'scrapped' altogether?

These and other questions of this kind are catalysts for this chapter, because they beg answers about the nature and effects of work practices and how they might be changed through technical reflection.

In this chapter I review information connected directly to technical reflection. I explain some of the reasons why this process is used for specific purposes and why it creates different outcomes in terms of knowledge of and practical answers to clinical problems. To do this, I step you through the relationships between empirical knowledge and the scientific method, and how the process for technical reflection fits with these ideas. I describe the connections between technical reflection and evidence-based practice and suggest that the two process are highly complementary.

151

I was keen to include technical reflection in this book, because I consider that it has been missing from texts on the subject thus far. Therefore, I justify the inclusion of technical reflection based on its validity as a form of knowledge and the usefulness of it for clinical practice. The process of technical reflection I have created is an eclectic approach, borrowing from Bandman and Bandman's (1995) view of scientific reasoning and the functions of critical thinkers, the features of critical thinking and thinkers described by van Hooft et al. (1995), and the problem-solving steps of the nursing process (Wilkinson 1996). The chapter provides an exercise in technical reflection and gives an example of how it has been used by a reflective practitioner.

REVIEW OF PREVIOUS IDEAS

As this relies on information given earlier in this book, I suggest that you revisit Chapters 1 and 6. However, as background to this chapter, I reiterate some essential points, which are connected directly to technical reflection.

Before you can practise technical reflection, you need to know some of the reasons why this process is used for specific purposes and why it creates specific outcomes in terms of knowledge of, and practical answers to, clinical problems. Therefore, you need to understand the relationships between empirical knowledge and the scientific method, and how the process for technical reflection fits with these ideas. What I am giving you is an explanation of epistemology, which you may remember is the study of how knowledge is generated and validated. Because there are so many ways of considering knowledge, there are actually many epistemologies. This description is a brief account of how a certain kind of knowledge is created and shown to be 'truthful' and useful.

Empirical knowledge is generated and tested through 'the scientific method'. It is called empirical because it rests on evidence from direct observation. The scientific method claims to be *the* method of knowledge-generation and validation, to the point that it has taken the word *scientia*, which means knowledge in general, and has applied it specifically to an epistemological method, which is actually only one of many ways of finding and checking 'truth' claims. Great success in creating knowledge, and the increased need for technology in the last 200 years or so, may have given the proponents of the scientific method confidence in it as the yardstick against which all other epistemological methods should be measured. The scientific method has been and continues to be very successful, because it uses strict criteria for setting up its enquiry and judging its truthfulness through rigorous and systematic measures including reliability, validity, and control and manipulation of variables.

Through the scientific method, data are quantified to demonstrate the degree of statistical significance in cause and effect relationships. In other words, information is converted into a form which can be measured and counted, so that it is possible to predict mathematically that the occurrence and behaviour of a phenomenon are significant, and not just happening by chance. To achieve this kind of predictive ability, scientific knowledge is rendered as free as possible from the distorting influences of people, who may skew the results with their prejudices, intentions and emotions. To avoid subjectivity of this kind, empirical researchers demand objectivity, meaning they strive to ensure that there is no involvement of prejudices, intentions and emotions in the conduct of the project. In summary, the scientific method creates empirical knowledge which can claim to be predictive and generalisable with some confidence that the conclusions are truthful, real, trustworthy and not just happening by chance.

The new or amended knowledge outcomes are achieved using the scientific method mainly through rational deductive thinking processes, which move systematically from broad to focused inferences. Scientific reasoning refers to a certain kind of rational argument, which underlies 'the scientific method'. The scientific approach to reasoning is to state a problem, give a preliminary hypothesis setting out the expected relationships between variables, collect more facts in order to formulate an hypothesis, deduce further consequences, test those consequences, and finally apply the findings to confirm or disconfirm the hypothesis (Bandman and Bandman 1995). Scientific reasoning provides a systematic approach to working through complex problems in an objective manner designed to keep the inquirer on track and to provide a means whereby other people can use a similar process to test whether the results can be replicated.

In Chapter 1, I discussed critical thinking, which is the

ability to think in a systematic and rational way. Scientific reasoning is aligned closely with critical thinking, in that the two thinking processes share many characteristics and often lead to similar outcomes. Critical thinking is essential for safe clinical practice and, according to many authors, rationality is its first requirement (Bandman and Bandman 1995; van Hooft, Gillam and Byrnes 1995; Wilkinson 1996). However, some authors stress that critical thinking is not just about rationality and emotional detachment for intellectual 'purity'. Even though van Hooft et al. (1995: 6–7) are keen to define the first important element of critical thinking as rational thinking, they emphasise that it is practical as well as theoretical—that it is conducive to dialogue and that it includes empathy and sensitive perception. They also describe critical thinkers as committed, self-aware and sympathetic to the commitments of others. The addition of practicality, dialogue, empathy and sensitivity in critical thinking, and self-aware and altruistic features in critical thinkers, gives critical thinking a 'human touch' that elevates it above a pure exercise of scientific rationality as described previously in this section. Even so, critical thinking borders on scientific reasoning because of its emphasis on rationality and scientific reasoning.

Earlier in this book I introduced you to the work of Jurgen Habermas. Although his philosophy can be dense conceptually, there has been a trend in the 1980s and 1990s to apply Habermas's work to practical areas such as curriculum (Mezirow 1981). Habermas is of interest to us as practitioners, because he had important things to say about the interests people have in their work, communication and power relations. When we consider technical reflection, we are focusing on what he had to say about work and procedures.

In Habermas's view (1972), technical interest in work creates 'instrumental action' through which people control and manipulate their environments. This means that people work with intention, so that by keeping a hold on situations they can achieve what they want. Therefore, people act in accordance with technical rules to generate empirical knowledge. In other words, they figure out the best ways of creating and following procedural steps in technical situations and claim that their results have been achieved through systematic and direct observation.

For nurses and midwives, technical interest is associated

with task-related competence, such as clinical procedures. You can see immediately that this is another way of talking about empirical knowledge, rationality, the scientific method, critical thinking and problem-solving. The scientific method's influence on empirical knowledge is apparent in daily practice because nurses and midwives have technical interest in their work. Many innovations and evidence-based adaptations in nursing and midwifery have been possible because of empirical knowledge, gained through empirical research, using processes I have described previously. Technical reflection fits into this discussion because I am suggesting that it is a way for you to integrate ways of thinking to allow you to adapt present procedures to better ones. You may also be able to predict likely outcomes for similar procedures and improve many work practices through objective and systematic lines of enquiry.

There has been a trend in the 1990s to speak of evidence-based nursing and midwifery (Pearson et al. 1997; Shorten and Wallace 1997). This is another way of saying that practice needs to be based on research findings rather than on rituals, traditions, whims and unfounded beliefs about what should be done in certain situations. If you have been practising for some time now, you can probably remember how nursing or midwifery procedures have changed over time. For example, in nursing you may have witnessed the transition from 'double nursing' of patients post myocardial infarction, to getting them out of bed and ambulating as soon as possible. In midwifery, you may have changed from undertaking 'peri' washes of bedfast women to encouraging them to ambulate to the bathroom to attend to their own perineum showers. At times, you may have wondered whether what you were doing was working at all and whether you had any technical justification for doing it. The evidence-based movement in nursing and midwifery is testing the validity of long-standing procedures such as the timing of ambulation, and it is seeking to replace old untested and unproven approaches with newer research-based ones.

CREATING THE PROCESS

I base the inclusion of the technical reflection in this book on its validity as a form of knowledge and its usefulness for clinical practice. I have described my support of empirical knowledge and technical reflection in this chapter and in Chapters 1 and 6. Rather than labour the point too severely, I suggest that you refer to those parts of this book. I will say at this point, however, that having decided on the legitimacy of using Habermas's work to describe all three forms of reflection, writing about technical reflection presented by far the greatest challenges for me personally.

I am known as a qualitative researcher and a supporter of finding meaning in life and practice through words and language. Even so, I can see the need for different types of inquiry based on the questions that are posed as conceptual challenges and puzzles. I have been concerned for some time that the critiques of science have laid bare the bones of the scientific method and have caused it to hurt from the sustained critique of scholars and philosophers. Even as I say this, however, I am aware that I do not need to defend empirical knowledge, because in some circles it is alive, well and as dominant as ever as *the* paradigm of inquiry. In other words, I wish that some researchers and ethics committee members were as conversant with and accepting of the forms and uses of qualitative research as they are with quantitative approaches.

What I am trying to express here is my belief in a need for balance in the ways of knowing and the legitimacy of them all for different purposes. This is why I included technical reflection in this book, to include processes that favour and support rationality in working through issues inherent in work procedures. I am not aware of any other attempts to do this in the literature on reflective practice specifically, although this area has been managed tangentially in texts on critical thinking, problem-solving and decision-making (Wilkinson 1996). So I hope you find this chapter insightful and helpful practically.

Having decided that technical reflection was important, I was then left with the problem of creating a process. I decided to take an eclectic approach, which basically means that I have borrowed from a number of sources. The technical reflective processes I describe in this chapter are based on Bandman and Bandman's (1995) view of scientific reasoning and the functions of critical thinkers, the features of critical thinking and thinkers described by van Hooft et al. (1995), and the problem-solving steps of the nursing process (Wilkinson 1996).

I have combined the thinking of all these authors so that the effects of their work can be augmented through technical reflection. Taken together, they also present a fairly balanced view of critical thinking by admitting human features such as dialogical relationships, intuition, empathy and sensitive perception. As nursing and midwifery are human disciplines, technical reflection must be based in the human condition, while it attends to developing rational arguments though applying the principles of scientific reasoning.

Important points to note

I must repeat a few very important points at this juncture. Although I consider that scientific reasoning has a clear and distinctive purpose in generating and validating empirical knowledge, this is not necessarily the case with critical thinking. In other words, critical thinking has wide applications and it may be helpful in any of the forms of reflection described in this book. However, I think that critical thinking is most likely to be useful when you are raising questions in your practice about technicalities related to the form and usefulness of your work procedures.

I also made the point previously that technical reflection may be used as a process in itself when you are working alone or with colleagues through observation and critical thinking, or it may be used in conjunction with a research project based on scientific reasoning. If clinical questions and issues are complex, technical reflection may accompany empirical research projects, which are based on reliability, validity, and control and manipulation of variables. The technical reflection thus instigated produces objective data that can be quantified to demonstrate the degree of statistical significance in cause and effect relationships. It is also possible that technical reflection could become part of mixed methodology research, such as an action research project which uses empirical methods to examine 'X' procedure as part of a larger collaborative group process.

Alternatively, if a question posed as a reflective task is less complex and does not require a research project *per se*, technical reflection alone can lead to answers based on observation and sound arguments that incorporate rational aspects of critical thinking. I am keen to keep you focused on manageable tasks in this book so you can experience immediate success, and for that reason I will not guide you through a research structure and process. This can be found in other books written specifically for research purposes such as Crookes and Davies (1998), LoBiondo and Haber (1994) or Roberts and Taylor (1998). Instead, I guide you through a process in which you raise a specific question about a clinical problem and you use an amalgam of processes and features adapted from Bandman and Bandman (1995), van Hooft et al. (1995) and Wilkinson (1996) to practise technical reflection.

In some cases, and at a later stage of your development as a reflective practitioner, you may require further validation of your thinking processes and move towards setting up a formal research project which can assess the relationship between variables of interest. Alternatively, the answers you acquire through a process of technical reflection may be sufficient for the work problems as presented. You need to exercise caution in determining whether the clinical problem was focused, analysed and resolved sufficiently by technical reflection alone. If there is any doubt as to whether the information generated is sufficient and effective, you may need to consider extending your reflections into a formal research project.

THE PROCESS OF TECHNICAL REFLECTION

In this section I present a process to assist you in using technical reflection in thinking about issues relating to a clinical procedure. In Chapter 3 I suggested many different methods for reflecting, and emphasised that these methods may be used alone or in combination to assist you in letting your thoughts flow during reflective processes. I also suggested that reflection does not have to be a solo effort. If you work better in groups, you can enlist a team or committee and go through reflective processes collaboratively. You may find that one 'run through' by yourself is a good idea, even if it just helps you get your thoughts together before a clinical meeting. Also, once you know how the process works, you can guide your colleagues through it, using this book as a reference.

This process encourages you to reflect on issues which require rational thinking for specific problems, but which do not require protracted work to solve them, such as in empirical research projects.

Using the method(s) of your choice, reflect on the following questions. Respond as carefully as you can, making sure that you attend to every step along the way. Use as many words as necessary to explain your position thoroughly, but keep to the point, so that you do not cloud the issue with extraneous information.

Think of a practice or procedure that has been established for some time, the value of which you have cause to question. I do not want to influence your choice of procedure by giving examples, so I will refer to it as 'Procedure X'.

Assessing and planning

In this part of the process, you set up the premises for rational thinking, by making an initial assessment of the problem and by planning for the development of an argument.

- What is Procedure X?
- Why is Procedure X done?
- How is Procedure X done?
- When is Procedure X done?
- What are the outcomes of Procedure X?
- Why do you believe that Procedure X is of questionable value?
- How do you propose to amend Procedure X?

From your responses to the previous questions, state the problem, giving a preliminary hypothesis about the expected relationships between the variables you have identified. If you are unable to state an hypothesis at this point you may need to spend more time assessing the problem, and you may need to collect more facts related to Procedure X.

- What words and language are associated commonly with Procedure X?

- Why are certain words and language associated commonly with Procedure X?
- Is there any evidence of misuse of words and language in Procedure X?
- Could the words and language associated commonly with Procedure X be stated differently?
- What nursing or midwifery problems are associated with Procedure X?

Implementing

In this part of the process, you develop an argument by analysing the issues and assumptions operating in the situation.

- What arguments are made to support the continuation of Procedure X in its present form?
- What nursing or midwifery assumptions underlie the support of Procedure X in its present form?
- What premises support the argument for Procedure X in its present form?
- Do these premises follow logically to provide sound conclusions?
- If not, why not?
- What inferences have been made and in what ways are they plausible, in supporting Procedure X in its present form?

Now is the time to formulate and clarify your own beliefs about Procedure X as stated in your hypothesis.

- What arguments are made to support the discontinuation of Procedure X in its present form?
- What nursing or midwifery assumptions underlie the opposition to Procedure X in its present form?
- On what premises are these arguments for opposing Procedure X in its present form based?
- Do these premises follow logically to provide sound conclusions?
- If not, why not?
- What inferences have been made and in what ways

are they plausible, in opposing Procedure X in its present form?

To test the consequences of the position that Procedure X is of questionable value in its present form, you need to implement some changes, or 'apply the findings' of rational deliberation in the practices associated with Procedure X. The changes would need to based on the results of rational discussion and decision-making, but they might include factors such as the time of day, the frequency of the procedure, preparations for Procedure X, the sequence of the method, and activities following Procedure X.

Evaluating

In this part of the process, you review the problem in light of all the information gained through the process of technical reflection.

- What information has been gained to date through implementing the technical reflection process?
- In what ways can you verify, corroborate and justify claims, beliefs, conclusions, decisions and actions taken in this process?
- What are the reasons for your beliefs and conclusions regarding this issue?
- What are your value judgments about this issue?
- To what extent can you claim that the conclusions you have reached are sound?
- What other possible consequences may transpire due to the conclusions reached by this process?

Make a succinct statement to either confirm or disconfirm the hypothesis as stated at the outset of this process.

The outcomes of technical reflection can be immediate, if the process has been shared with, and the findings endorsed by, the key people who are in a position to influence and ratify nursing and midwifery practice. You may find that this process has many applications. For example, you could use technical reflection to think critically through your own practice issues, or it could be used in groups as, say, a guide for a clinical policy and practice meeting agenda, as an outline for analysing technical issues in ward/unit clinical discussions and/or as part of the methods of formal research. In whatever situations you use it, technical reflection has the potential for allowing you to think critically and reason scientifically, so that you can critique and adapt present procedures to better ones as necessary. You may also be able to predict likely outcomes for similar procedures and improve many work practices through objective and systematic lines of enquiry.

AN EXAMPLE OF TECHNICAL REFLECTION

In this section I provide an example of technical reflection, based on a story Michael wrote in his journal. Although Michael's story is not about a technical procedure as such, it is about an administrative practice of understaffing the night shift. Michael needed to use critical thinking to make sense of the technical aspects of the situation and to ensure that, in the future, ill patients are cared for adequately during the night hours.

In providing this example, I used the questions listed in the technical reflection process above. I have left the practitioner's account as he wrote it to retain its authenticity and to demonstrate to you the need to trust that your own writing style is useful for reflection. The tangle of tenses, abbreviations and other grammatical glitches are typical of the way practitioners speak and write, so they have been retained in Michael's story to maintain the authenticity of his account.

Lorna C was a woman in her 70s, ex-smoker with COAD who has had a radical neck dissection. Her respiratory management post-op has been quite a handful. We came on duty at 9.30 p.m. at night to find that Lorna has been troubled by a cough and is thought to maybe be brewing a chest infection. No great surprise given her history. Antibiotics cannot be started until a sputum specimen is obtained and of course the staff have been too busy.

When we first see Lorna she is sleeping soundly (no surprise as she has not slept the previous night). Her chest sounds dreadful as it always does but there is no cough—obs are stable.

We are now stuck with how to manage her over-night. The choice is to let her sleep and give her active chest physio every time she wakes. This holds until 0430 when Lorna wakes feeling very short of breath. O_2 saturation on 6L/min of O_2 is 78%. Listening to her chest the crackles have gone to mid-zones and temp is 38.5. I ring the physician who is notorious for not giving clear orders in the middle of the night. I hit the jackpot, he seems to cotton on to what I am saying—probable situation pulmonary oedema on top of pneumonia. Orders—turn off IV (yes), get blood cultures (yes), IV Lasix (yes), insert IDC (yes). He is right on the ball. Welcome back to clinical practice—she is shut down peripherally so I take my first stab at a patient for blood in about four years and I am virtually going in blind—got it on the second try (there has to be some benefit to working at the sexually trans-mitted disease clinic and getting all those blood samples).

Next the Lasix—that's easy. IDC on a female—first time. I realise that I've actually retained quite a few clinical skills that I thought were long gone.

Unfortunately Lorna does not respond to Lasix and air entry remains poor and O_2 sats low. I ring *physician again, this is where the true colours show. More Lasix (yes), increased, O_2 (yes), but only a temporary relief. Blood gases at 0700hrs (<u>wrong</u>)— what do I do to keep this patient from arresting for the next 1.25 hours?*

I try to think of what rationale you would use for holding off on the blood gases, unfortunately the only one I can think of is that it allows the physician more sleep.

The patient is tired but lasts till blood gases are done at 0700hrs. These are what we expect, and she is transferred to a major hospital ICU within the hour.

While some of this has been pure frustration, e.g. sitting on critically ill patients in a ward environment, the fact that I have retained some skills I thought would be gone is a bit of a buzz.

APPLYING A TECHNICAL REFLECTION PROCESS

In this section I analyse Michael's story about Lorna by applying it to a technical reflection process. Michael expresses the clinical situation mainly in an objective style, and he uses rationality in determining Lorna's condition and how he should act in relation to it. In applying Michael's story to a technical reflection process, certain facts and assumptions surface, and an argument can be developed to defend future practice.

In Michael's story about Lorna, the clinical problem is how to manage a critically ill patient throughout the night and early morning hours, to balance her need for rest and lung secretion drainage.

Assessing and planning

In this part of the process, you set up the premises for rational thinking, by making an initial assessment of the problem and by planning for the development of an argument.

The 'procedure' or clinical task at hand was to manage Lorna's shortness of breath when she awoke at 0430 hours, so Michael performed a blood gas saturation and listened to her chest. He then phoned the physician with the results of the assessment; the physician directed Michael to turn off the intravenous infusion, obtain blood cultures, give intravenous Lasix, and insert an indwelling catheter.

In testing the blood gas saturation and listening to Lorna's chest, Michael assessed the degree of lung congestion. In informing the physician, Michael requested medical assistance to relieve Lorna's dyspnoea. In following the physician's directions, Michael instituted measures to relieve pulmonary congestion.

The outcomes of the interventions were not successful immediately, as evidenced by the lack of diuresis, poor air entry and low blood oxygen saturation. In view of these indicators, Michael rang the physician again. This time he was directed to administer more Lasix and oxygen, but to repeat the blood gases at 0700 hours.

Michael could not work out the physician's rationale for withholding the blood gas measurement for 1.25 hours, although he suspected that it was to allow the physician more time to sleep. Michael's immediate problem was to prevent Lorna from having a cardiac arrest until he could check her blood gas levels at 0700 hours. When the results were available at the designated time, they indicated Lorna's critical condition and she was transferred to a major Intensive Care Unit within the hour.

Although Michael's story ends here and he made no suggestions about how to amend the problem of managing patients such as Lorna who are critically ill on the night duty shift, I have imagined the responses he might make to the questions in the technical reflection process.

The clinical problem is the management of critically ill patients during the night shift when physicians need to be woken from their sleep to give directions for medical care. A preliminary hypothesis of the situation is that meeting the needs of critically ill patients on the night shift is related directly to the provision by the hospital of better resources and to improvements in nurse–doctor communication.

The words and language associated commonly with the care of critically ill patients are objective and instrumental. For example, Michael wrote: 'Lorna wakes feeling very short of breath. O_2 saturation on 6L/min of O_2 is 78%. Listening to her chest the crackles have gone to mid-zones and temp is 38.5 . . . probable situation pulmonary oedema on top of pneumonia. Orders—turn off IV, get blood cultures, IV Lasix, insert IDC.'

Objective and instrumental words and language are associated commonly with the care of critically ill patients, because they convey the need for a non-emotional response, directed towards quick and effective management.

In expressing himself and his memory of the situation, Michael used certain words and phrases which demonstrated his value judgments and assumptions about the likely behaviour of the physician. For example, he wrote: 'I ring the physician who is notorious for not giving clear orders in the middle of the night. I hit the jackpot, he seems to cotton on to what I am saying—probable situation pulmonary oedema on top of pneumonia. Orders—turn off IV (yes), get blood cultures (yes), IV Lasix (yes), insert IDC (yes).'

The use of this language in relation to the physician is probably related to Michael's anxiety at having the responsibility for dealing with a critically ill patient in the early morning hours. The words he wrote may have been different if Michael had been in a position to speak with the physician as an equal negotiating the care of the patient.

The nursing problems associated with caring for critically ill patients in the early morning hours, and having to rely on physicians' phone orders, are that the nurses do all the assessment, feel great anxiety for the patient's sake, and are caught in the bind of needing to adhere to the conventions of the nurse–doctor relationship. Michael was playing the 'nurse–doctor game', because he did all the work and handed the results over to the doctor to take the initiative and credit for care. In other words, Michael did all of the physical assessment of Lorna, and although he knew the problem was pulmonary oedema, he did not deign to diagnose as he felt he was not in a position to do so. Therefore, even though Michael gave the physician all of the information he needed to decide on treatment, he did not question the timing of the follow-up blood gas estimation. In effect, he felt he had no option but to accept the doctor's directions, even though he suspected the physician had nonaltruistic motives for giving them.

Implementing

In this part of the process, you develop an argument by analysing the issues and assumptions operating in the situation.

An argument to support the continuation of the present procedure for managing critically ill patients in the early morning hours rests on economic and personal reasons. Some hospitals cannot afford to have medical staff on call and available within the facility. The costs involved in maintaining regular on-site medical assistance are prohibitive, in view of the fact that the number of actual emergencies in a twelve-month period is relatively low. Also, the private hospital system ensures that patients have access to the care of their own physician. Taken to its logical conclusion, this would mean that all physicians with patients admitted overnight would need to sleep in the hospital in case patients deteriorated unexpectedly and required immediate medical assistance. Physicians are not willing to commit this much of their personal time to their work, based on the likelihood that problems may arise. If patients become critically ill, the doctor can be contacted by phone to give the necessary orders, based on the objective evidence of the patient's condition as supplied by the attending nurse. Therefore, the present procedure for managing patients during the night shift is adequate. In the matter of nurse–doctor communication, there is not a problem. Doctors are in charge of patient care. Nurses are subordinate to doctors and it is their duty to do as doctors order.

The nursing assumptions underlying the present procedures for managing critically ill patients in the early morning hours are that nurses are prepared professionally to cope with all contingencies, that doctors are responsible for medical management and that there is a convention of managing critically ill patients during the night shift which works under most conditions.

The premises of the arguments supporting the present procedures for managing critically ill patients in the early morning hours are that the facility's physical resources are adequate, the nursing staff are capable of monitoring and reporting changes in patients' conditions, they can request that a doctor attend in a medical emergency, and they have the phone back-up of physicians if it is required.

These premises follow logically to provide sound conclusions if the facilities and the nursing staff and physicians are operating at peak performance. The argument falls down if one patient dies due to lack of performance on the part of the staff concerned.

The inferences in the argument for supporting the present procedures for managing critically ill patients in the early morning hours are that the system presently in place works because nurses and physicians know their roles and attend to them professionally. This is a plausible argument, even though the complexities of nursing and medical practice may test these inferences from time to time.

On Michael's behalf, I made a preliminary hypothesis that meeting the needs of critically ill patients on the night shift is related directly to the provision by the hospital of better resources and to improvements in nurse–doctor communication.

My argument to oppose continuation of the present procedures for managing critically ill patients in the early morning hours is based on their failure to cater to the needs of patients and on the need to revise the economic and personal constraints that do not permit more effective care. Lorna and other like cases show that nurses are carrying undue pressure and responsibility due to lack of on-site medical assistance and the inadequacies of nurse–doctor communication.

Economic constraints are the most frequently cited reason for insufficient nursing staff on shifts, even though limited numbers of nurses working with critically ill patients mean that there is a greater chance of difficulties arising. Although hospitals are run as businesses, they should value people over profits. Therefore, if the hospital is committed to patient care, as it espouses, it will direct dollars to ensuring that all shifts are adequately staffed by nurses and that doctors receive the necessary inducements to ensure their cooperation in patient care.

The personal aspects of communication between nurses and doctors require attention, given that they are rooted deeply in historical, cultural, political, economic and social variables, which have caused the nurse–doctor relationship to evolve in certain ways. Nurses and doctors need to negotiate more direct ways of talking to one another, so that they can speak frankly about their assessment of patients' situations and the likely success of management strategies.

The nursing assumptions underlying this position are that nurses become expert in their practice, and they know what is happening to patients when vital signs change as signs and symptoms manifest. Sometimes a patient's condition deteriorates beyond that which can be expressed in medical terms—that is, the nurse has an intuitive sense that treatment will not be effective even before the vital signs change. Statements of intuition are not prized by many doctors, who prefer scientific reasoning alone, with no expression of empathy or sensitive perception. Being with the patient means that nurses are in a first-hand position to notice responses to treatment and to adjust the care as necessary. The traditional roles and responsibilities of nurses and doctors and the relationships they have evolved over time weigh against them treating each other as equals and carrying on logical and reasonable discussions about patient management based on mutual respect and trust.

The premise for this argument is that the clinical expertise of nurses is established and that it needs to be acknowledged by doctors. This does not mean that nurses should be responsible for direct patient management, but rather that they should speak more directly to doctors about their interpretations of what physicians direct them to do. Therefore, nurses need to claim their expertise and be confident in asserting it, so that they do not perpetuate their own subordination in the nurse–doctor relationship. The premises follow logically to provide sound conclusions if the basic nature of the nurse–doctor relationship can be changed to allow for more direct discussion about patient management.

The inferences that have been made in suggesting a more direct form of nurse–doctor communication are that these professionals are adults, who are capable of mature communication. Although nurses and doctors have different backgrounds in terms of eduction and training, they are involved actively in patient care, and they approach it from unique perspectives. Although communication patterns over time have set up a superior–subordinate relationship in terms of power between doctors and nurses, there is common ground on which to build mutual respect and trust and direct communication about patient management. This requires some assertion on the part of nurses and some listening on the part of doctors, but if nurses can find voice and become confident that they are being heard, doctors will realise that nurses are integral and relatively equal in deciding the best possible strategies for patient care.

To test the consequences of the position that meeting the needs of ill patients on the night shift is related directly to the provision by the hospital of better resources and to improvements in nurse–doctor communication, rational discussion and decision-making over a protracted period would need to occur. Practitioners and representatives of the hospital system would need to set up discussion about the resources needed to support the care of critically ill patients during the night shift. Nurses and doctors would need to work systematically through the factors that determine their relationship to build new relationships based on respect and trust, which favour more direct communication about patient management. Neither of these two aims is a simple matter. A great deal of technical reflection on the part of all the people concerned would be necessary to make a difference in this situation. I suppose this is why many situations do not change. The people involved get a sense of the complexity of the situation and do not make attempts to change what they think is unchangeable.

Evaluating

In this part of the process, you review the problem in light of all the information gained through the process of technical reflection. As this is a situation which has not been acted upon, I can only imagine what technical reflection might look like if a positive outcome was possible. Accordingly, I project a positive outcome, using as a guide the questions listed previously in the technical reflection process.

After meetings between practitioners and representatives of the hospital, the resources needed for the management of critically ill patients in the early morning hours were identified as people resources in the form of extra staff. Lorna's dilemma was intensified by the lack of a sputum result and the subsequent prescription of antibiotics. 'Being busy' was cited as the reason for the inability of the previous nursing shift to obtain a sputum specimen, and the lack of antibiotics related directly to the development of chest congestion. The hospital administrators agreed to roster an extra nurse on afternoon shifts, with the expressed purpose of taking a case load to relieve the usual pressures of evening shifts, and to ensure that diagnostic tests are done and specimens are collected to allow treatment to proceed.

I would also like to pretend that the nurses and doctors got together and talked through all the personal, historical, cultural, political, economic and social reasons why their relationships have evolved as they have, but even I can't stretch my imagination that far! Pulling apart and restructuring the nurse–doctor relationship will take a long time of concentrated effort between both parties and I can suggest no easy quick fix suggestions. However, as promised I will project a positive outcome.

In a regular clinical case meeting between health professionals in the hospital, Lorna's case was described by Michael from his perspective in charge of her nursing care. The physician was present and he recognised his role in the situation. Michael's version of the events lacked the extra words he wrote that showed his frustration with the physician and his concern that the phone orders would probably not be clear. A nurse present at the meeting asked Michael to retell the story, this time inserting the way he was feeling at the time and why. She then asked Michael to tell the group about the problems he sees with the present procedures for managing critically ill patients in the early morning hours and what strategies he could suggest to amend them. Michael explained his hypothesis that meeting the needs of critically ill patients on the night shift is related directly to the provision by the hospital of better resources and to improvements in nurse–doctor communication. He then provided the argument described previously in the technical reflection process.

To verify his beliefs and conclusions in the matter, Michael cited the comparisons between Lorna's case and other clinical situations in which there had been difficulty with phone directions. He also admitted that the nurses involved often felt unable or unwilling to assert themselves in discussions with physicians about patient management. Other nurses present described their own experiences and corroborated Michael's experience and argument.

Michael's beliefs and conclusions on this issue were founded on the need for optimal patient safety and for professional security of nurses working without immediate and 'on the spot' medical assistance in the early morning hours. There was also a belief in the expertise of nurses and a desire to see better lines of direct communication in which nurses feel able and willing to assert themselves in negotiating patient management with physicians who are not present to take in all the cues manifesting in the patient's illness.

Michael's value judgments in this issue related to his previous experience of unsatisfactory phone conversations with physicians and a working knowledge that nurses play subordinate roles to doctors and are not valued by them. Michael also made a value judgment that the timing for the blood gas analysis was not related to Lorna's welfare, but to the physician's need for sleep. Michael made a value judgment that the physician was acting selfishly and did not have Lorna's best interests in mind.

Michael reached sound conclusions in his argument based on this and his previous experiences, which he documented objectively and systematically. He owned up to his feelings of frustration and reworded his argument in terms which stated the facts of the matter, showing the relationship between events that added up to unsatisfactory procedures for the management of critically ill patients in the early morning hours.

Although the conclusions reached in this case related to the specific consequences of an extra nurse on evening shifts and the beginning of open dialogue with physicians, other possible consequences could involve a formal overview of other incidents in which nurse–doctor relationships could be improved for the benefit of patient care.

After a process of individual and group technical reflection, the hypothesis was confirmed that meeting the needs of ill patients on the night shift is related directly to the provision by the hospital of better resources and to improvements in nurse–doctor communication.

SUMMARY

Questions about clinical procedures can be answered quickly and effectively through technical reflection. In this chapter I reviewed some previous information given in this book, connected directly to technical reflection. I explained some of the reasons why technical reflection is used for specific purposes and why it creates practical answers to clinical problems. To do this, I reviewed the relationships between empirical knowledge and the scientific method, and how the process for technical reflection fits with these ideas. I described the connections between technical reflection and evidence-based practice and suggested that the two processes are highly complementary.

I included technical reflection in this book on its basis as a form of knowledge generation, which is useful for clinical practice. I described the process of technical reflection as an amalgam of Bandman and Bandman's (1995) view of scientific reasoning and the functions of critical thinkers, the features of critical thinking and thinkers described by van Hooft et al. (1995), and the problem-solving steps of the nursing process (Wilkinson 1996). The chapter provided an exercise in technical reflection and gave an example of how it could be used by a reflective practitioner. I hope that you find technical reflection useful in your work.

8

Practical reflection

- Why do I strive to be a perfect practitioner?
- How am I affected by patients' pain and suffering?
- Why is interpersonal communication at work so complex?
- How can I be more therapeutic in my interpersonal relationships at work?

These questions are all about creating a better understanding of what it is like to experience and to make sense out of living a life in relation to other people and events. Sometimes your reflection will be about your own personal and professional growth issues, the nature of phenomena such as the experience of illness, the meaning of events of clinical importance, and the dynamics and significance of interpersonal relationships. When this is the case, you will find that practical reflective processes will help you to interpret the communicative aspects of your work setting and the people within it.

In this chapter I will review some of the content of Chapter 6 to remind you of the assumptions on which practical reflection is based, before I guide you through a reflective exercise and present some stories from Carol's experience.

REVIEW OF PREVIOUS IDEAS

In Chapter 6 I described practical reflection in relation to interpretive knowledge and practical interests. Practical reflection is related to interpretive knowledge, because it centres on people and values their perceptions of their life experiences and their ability to communicate them. People communicate through language, symbols, ceremonies, rituals, art forms and other behavioural practices. Of all the means of communication, the main way of making and sharing meaning is through speaking words that convey ideas, concepts, theories, propositions and so on. One of the most important reasons for language and interpersonal discussion is the communication of human experience, because people assign significance to what is happening within their own bodies and lives, and to similar concerns of other people. Practical reflection focuses on human experience and communication to make sense out of these phenomena through experiencing, interpreting and learning from them.

Interpretive knowledge centres on people, because of their perceptions of their life experiences and their ability to communicate them. The underlying concepts of interpretive knowledge include interpersonal understanding through attention to people's lived experience, context and subjectivity.

Lived experience means knowing what it is like to live a life in a particular time, place and set of circumstances. It involves the interpretation of experiences which make up the fabric of human existence, once they have been opened up to reflection. It is only through reflection that people can make sense of their lived experiences, because time must elapse—whether it is moments or years—to sort through the meaning of experiences. Daily life is always moving forward towards the next experience and it is so easy to get caught up in it and to just let it happen. If you think of what it is like to be a human, the movement forward of life is within a body in a social world, and in respect to everything which occurs as part of living. In a sense, we are propelled forward by the prospect of tomorrow, and we cannot help but accumulate experiences along the way. This being so, there is a need to make sense of lived experience, in order to prepare for further forward movement by reflecting on what has happened, why and how, so that we can learn in the present and project these new insights into the future. Therefore, lived experience is an important concept in understanding interpretive knowledge and how it fits into practical reflection.

Context means all of the features of the time and place in which people find themselves, in which they locate their lives. If you think now of your context, how would you describe it? My context presently is that I am living at the turn of the twenty-first century on the far North Coast of New South Wales. This is where I work as an academic and where I reside with my partner and son. My context is also described by my age, gender and social and political affiliations, such as my friends, colleagues and other relationships and my work and home interests. I could go on to describe more and more of my context and the more I describe, the broader and deeper my context would become. I cannot help but be connected to my context in all of its features, because I relate to it as part of myself and, in turn, it tells me who I am. Interpretive knowledge is explained in part by context because it situates people in their experiences and gives them some markers for making sense of their lives. This is also how it relates to practical reflection.

Subjectivity refers to the individual's sensing of inner and external events, which includes personal experiences and truths, that may or may not be like other people's subjective experiences and truths. In this book I am using the word 'subjectivity' in an uncomplicated way, which tries to avoid the tangle philosophical thought has put it into in trying to differentiate it from objectivity. In relation to interpretive knowledge, subjectivity is the means through which individuals sense phenomena inside and outside themselves. Therefore, it is a form of knowledge within the person as subject—that is, the person who relates towards objects of attention. Subjectivity is a part of interpretive knowledge, because it is created by the person as the knower, who makes sense of his or her experiences.

Intersubjectivity refers to how individuals take account of one another in the social world to make sense of their experiences. We tend to live in social circumstances and therefore we need to take account of other people and their experiences. Interpretive knowledge is formed in part by people in dialogue with one another, negotiating the sense they make out of experiences by sharing and contesting meaning in human communication.

In summary, interpretive knowledge emerges from the perspectives of people engaged actively in their lives and it includes and values what people feel and think. Judgments as to the usefulness and 'truthfulness' of the accounts are based on the relative indicators, such as the nature of lived experience, context and subjectivity.

In Chapter 6 I also introduced the idea of practical interest, derived from the work of Jurgen Habermas. To some extent, I have already linked practical interest and interpretive knowledge, but you may find further explanation useful at this point. Practical interest involves human interaction or 'communicative action', which involves reciprocal expectations about behaviour which are defined and understood by the people involved. In other words, and put into the negative if it did not exist, we would have no means of making sense of communication if we did not agree on what certain words and symbols mean. Through this lack of consensus, it follows that we would not have a common basis for agreeing on the relevant action needed in certain circumstances.

In a work setting, communicative action translates to something as familiar as the communication patterns that are set up by clinicians and the people with whom they come into contact. Communicative action in nursing or midwifery relates to agreeing on and acting upon shared communication norms and expectations. Social norms, or sets of expectations for behaviour, are created over time by people who are in consensus about what is expected in certain situations. The social norms are enforced through sanctions, which ensure that people recognise and honour their responsibilities in the reciprocal behaviour. Thus communicative action is a rich source of interest for practical reflection. As the main intentions of practical interests are to describe and explain human interaction, they are concerned with interpretation and explanation through practical reflection, which in turn creates interpretive knowledge.

ADAPTING THE PROCESS

When I turned my attention towards practical reflection, I knew that, in setting out a process, I could use and adjust some of the ideas I had been conversant with for some time.

I used an amalgam of different views on critical thinking and scientific reasoning to create a process for technical reflection, as I could not locate a pre-existing process under the umbrella of reflection *per se*. However, when I came to the task of putting forward a practical reflection process, I realised that this would involve adjustment of what has been used previously in the work of Smyth (1986a, 1986b) and Street (1991) as an interpretive beginning to what is essentially an emacipatory process.

Practical reflection is important in itself. As with technical reflection, I wanted to draw out the practical interests of clinicians into a form of reflection that could stand alone, or be used in combination with other forms of reflection. The reason for this is that there is immense value in reflecting for the purposes of interpreting and learning from work life. Although change may not be an explicit aim of practical reflection, it is still possible through new insights that follow from raised awareness.

In the process which follows, I have retained some of the questions used previously (Smyth 1986a, 1986b; Street 1991) but I have adjusted the language to fit an interpretive knowledge paradigm and I have presented the process as experiencing, interpreting and learning. Experiencing involves retelling a practice story so that you experience it again in as much detail as possible. Interpreting involves clarifying and explaining the meaning of a communicative action situation. Learning involves creating new insights and integrating them into your existing awareness and knowledge.

Important points to note

I cautioned previously that, while practical reflection is helpful, it has limitations in what it can offer you. Through the medium of language, practical reflection will help you to understand the interpersonal basis of human experiences and it will also offer you the potential for creating new knowledge which interprets the meaning of your lived experience, context and subjectivity. You can experience changes through practical reflection, although that is not its primary aim. The changes will be based on your raised awareness of the nature and effects of a wide range of communicative matters pertaining to your practice.

178

However, practical reflection will not offer you the objective means to observe and analyse work procedures through a scientific method, because it does not have an interest in instrumental action. Also, practical reflection will not give you a process for making a radical critique of the constraining forces and power influences within your work settings. The reason for this is that, although practical reflection can raise awareness through insights into communicative action, unlike emancipatory reflection, it does not have transformative action as its primary concern.

THE PROCESS OF PRACTICAL REFLECTION

At this point, you may find it helpful to refer to Chapter 3, in which I suggested some prerequisites for reflecting. There are many strategies for reflecting, which you can use alone or in combination. If you have been reading through this book sequentially, by now you will be equipped with some of the literature which affirms the usefulness of reflective practice and some stories from other nurses and midwives who have begun reflecting on their practice. You may also have undertaken a 'warm up' exercise, in which I encouraged you to think about the person and professional you are now in light of childhood memories and rules for living. In the previous chapter, you may have also applied technical reflective processes to procedural work requiring improvement through rational processes. We are now at the point at which it is time to reflect on some practice incidents which could benefit from practical reflection.

The focus of your stories is you. You are the focus if you are interested in gaining from new insights from your experiences. To some extent, life is an individual experience. Even with people you think you know well, you actually stand outside their life and experiences. Therefore, as you cannot really know what it is like to live their life, you are not really in a position to dictate the way that person experiences, interprets, explains or learns from his or her work or home life. In other words, in this process you need to begin with a resolve to 'mind your own business' and to 'attend to your own affairs'. If other people do likewise, there can be a collective effect, especially when like-minded people band together for collaborative action on common causes. However, in the first steps towards practical reflection, the responsibility resides with you. For this reason, all the responses you give to the questions posed in the process will be in relation to your own perceptions, valid only for your experiences.

In the exercise that follows, I would like you to reflect on your own work setting and practice, because these stories require you to be active and central to what is happening. You can use the process as a means of exploring any questions and concerns related to the interpersonal basis of your work experiences. When you have recorded one scenario, you can go on to reflect on as many as you choose. Although a daily reflective habit is excellent, if you can manage only one focused attempt each week that will be useful. You might find that your reflection is more of a matter of quality than quantity.

As I explained in Chapter 3, it is important to keep a compilation of all your reflections, because you will need them to compare your insights over time. They will show you your main issues and how you are working through them using reflective processes. So, here we go!

Think of an incident at work, in which you were undertaking your usual work activities involving interpersonal communication, that you felt did not go well. In other words, the situation did not develop the positive outcomes you had envisioned. Write your responses in your journal or record them through audio or video tape, ensuring that you can review your answers for later analysis.

Experiencing

Experiencing involves retelling a practice story so that you experience it again in as much detail as possible.

In this part of the process, it is important to recall the sights, sounds, smells, people and any other features which had bearing on the incident. It might help if you shut your eyes and take yourself back in your imagination to that time. Alternatively, you might like to begin the process by getting ready emotionally through creative means, such as by playing music, painting, poetry or any of the other strategies mentioned in Chapter 3. When you have a clear image of the situation, write down or represent creatively a full description of the experience. Refer to yourself in the first person, so that you remain engaged centrally and actively in the story. Let your thinking flow so that you portray your head image as faithfully as possible. Respond to the following questions to build up a thick description of the experience:

- What was happening?
- When was it happening?
- Where was it happening?
- Why was it happening?
- Who was involved?
- How were you involved?
- What was the setting like, in terms of its smells, sounds and sights?
- What were the outcomes of the situation?
- How did you feel honestly about the situation?

Let the reflection end when it exhausts itself, then review what you have written or represented in some other creative form. Compare the image in your head with your representation of the event. How do the image and the representation of the reflection compare? If the words or other means of creative expression do not do justice to your head image, go back and elaborate further to ensure that you have encapsulated the experience as well as you possibly can.

Interpreting

Interpreting involves clarifying and explaining the meaning of a communicative action situation.

You should have before you a fully descriptive scenario of situational and communicative aspects of your experience. To make sense of the story, you will need to revisit the account to locate yourself and the communication patterns that were set up with the other people. To find the communicative action features in the story, read the account or review the creative representation and ask yourself:

- What were my hopes for the practice outcomes in this story?
- How were my hopes related to my ideals of what constitutes 'good' practice?
- What are the sources in my life and work for my ideas and values for communicative aspects of my practice?
- In what ways do I embody them now in the way I communicate at work?
- What was my communicative role in this situation?
- To what extent did I achieve my communicative role?
- How did my interpretation of my role affect my relations with the people in the situation?
- What are the shared communication norms and expectations in this situation? (In other words, how did everyone else in the story interpret their roles and what did they seem to expect in the situation?)
- To what extent were social norms, or sets of expectations for behaviour, operating in this situation?
- What sanctions were in place to ensure that people in this situation recognised and honoured their responsibilities for maintaining socially approved reciprocal behaviour? (Remember, the sanctions or coercive measures may have been obvious (explicit) or hidden (implicit), but they nevertheless operated as ways of authorising and controlling the situation.)
- Were the usual communicative norms and sanctions altered in this situation?

Learning

Learning involves creating new insights and integrating them into your existing awareness and knowledge.

- What does this scenario tell me about my expectations of myself?

- What does this scenario tell me about my expectations of other people?
- What have I learned from this situation?
- What kinds of adaptations are possible in my work relationships?
- How do I fit these new insights into my present ways of regarding communicative action in my work?

Record your responses to these questions and discuss them with a critical friend. When you are ready, apply your new learning to your work situation.

In considering these questions, you are making an interpretation of human interactions in your practice. You will begin to see that, even though you are often at the centre of the action, you are certainly not the only person contributing to the situation. Human communication is complex and by looking at the relationships and shared norms you will raise your awareness about your own values and action, and how they relate to those held by other people. This means that you will have a greater understanding of your own communication patterns and those of the people with whom you work.

AN EXAMPLE OF PRACTICAL REFLECTION

In this section I will provide an example of practical reflection, based on a story Carol wrote in her journal. As far as possible, I will use the questions I listed in the practical reflection process above, although in some cases they may be irrelevant.

As I mentioned before, I have left the practitioners' accounts as they wrote them to retain their authenticity and to demonstrate the need to trust that your own writing style is useful for reflection. You will notice that Carol writes in brief sentences, which do not provide rich description; however, she is documenting her practice and opening it up to her own reflection.

Coming on in pm and taking over from a student midwife. Report taken and round of patients to check their status, introduce myself and plan the evening's activities.

Within five minutes patient came wanting discharge—she has twins. The student knew about it but hadn't even started discharge.

So I began because there was twins, double the paperwork, then they had clicky hips, more paperwork included. Midwives data collections forms ¥ 2.

Blue books, two sections ¥ 2 and found clicky hips documented four days previous.

Notification of abnormalities ¥ 2.

Then for Mum—usual antenatal card, D/C slip, also referral to community nurses for gaping wound. Needed referral phone call and then fax. Babies' clicky hips means ringing paediatrician, then to see orthopaedic specialist and ?hip brace.

I got hold of a different paediatrician and so we decided to get patient to come from (town X) to (town Y), half hour, this should have been done previously.

One and a half hours of paper work and script getting, referral, successful discharge. Hug on the way out for woman.

2nd patient. Student had tried to discharge another woman all day. She handed over to me to keep trying to ring a number which was not answering which would have contacted a woman who would come and get the girl to come take back to (town Z) (Koori girl). Previous night they had transport but no capsule and staff wouldn't let them go without proper security.

I thought if this transport couldn't be contacted

and the hospital may have been able to transport tomorrow as it was too late to organise this today. So the lady would just stay the night.

Then at 6pm an Aboriginal man came up and said they were ready to go so I went down with the appropriate paperwork, did a quick postnatal check and observations and talked a little bit and discharged the girl with a capsule and her own arranged transport.

Reflections

Junior staff possibly overwhelmed with procedures of discharge and paperwork, also student was English and not used to talking with Aboriginal patients.

Twin paperwork typical double paperwork. I filled out three pieces of paper for the same thing and because it was twins it was double this. Referrals and proper handover.

I question the validity of statistical collection of the neonatal abnormalities. The extra piece of paper has only been made aware to me recently— what about the four years worth of abnormalities (congenital terminations for abnormalities) has been large in number but no forms have gone in so large under-reporting.

Working cross-culturally. Did the student actually discuss discharge with the lady? Did the girl answer truthfully and what if we stopped trying to fix things and let the situation flow the resources of women and support of their families?

?? decreased discussion with patient because of differing communication expectations.

APPLYING A PRACTICAL REFLECTION PROCESS

The way in which Carol expresses her role in the clinical situation is in a short sentence, minimally descriptive style, but we can gain some appreciation of her experience. In applying Carol's story to a practical reflection process, I will use some of the information she has supplied in her 'reflections'; however, I will need to use 'creative licence' to extend the experience so that it can be helpful in assisting you to understand how to apply a practical reflection process to your work situations.

As this is not my experience, I can only hope to provide a commentary and raise some questions as a critical friend. I have read the account, but I have not had an opportunity to discuss this with Carol.

Experiencing

In this account, we are given some details about two patients for whom Carol cared in one day at work. In the first story, Carol received a handover from a student midwife, who had not started discharge arrangements for a mother with her twins. This resulted in a great deal of work for Carol, involving 'double the paperwork', the problem of the complex and lengthy process for discharging a baby with clicky hips, and a referral of the mother to the community nurses for care of a gaping wound.

Although there is sufficient detail in Carol's account to let me know what is happening, when and where, she does not provide extra information, such as a description of what the setting was like, in terms of its smells, sounds and sights, and how she honestly felt about the situation. I infer that Carol was not very pleased with the communicative action on a number of counts. I base this impression on my experience as a midwife and on the way Carol has identified certain people and listed the activities she had to undertake to manage a 'successful discharge'. Carol referred to 'a student midwife', who 'knew about it [the impending discharge] but hadn't even started discharge'. The list of activities demonstrated the amount of work which needed to be done. Although Carol did not share how she felt about the need for her to do this work, I infer that it was frustrating for her, because in her 'reflections' she wrote: '*Junior staff* possibly overwhelmed with procedures of discharge and paperwork' (my emphasis), and she also questioned 'the validity of statistical collection of the neonatal abnormalities'. Sometimes it is useful to let out your feelings about how a situation affects you, because you can acknowledge it to yourself and other people, and begin to see how events could be different.

The second account involved an Indigenous Australian woman, with whom there was inadequate communication about the need for a baby capsule in the car taking mother and child home. I infer that Carol was frustrated with how 'the student' managed this procedure. Carol wrote: 'Working cross-culturally. Did the student actually discuss discharge with the lady? Did the girl answer truthfully and what if we stopped trying to fix things and let the situation flow the resources of women and support of their families?' I do not know what emotions Carol felt in relation to experiencing these work incidents. It is possible that Carol may not have been frustrated and that I have made an incorrect inference in this situation. The point I am making is that each part of the process is important if the experience is to be described well enough to make some interpretation of it through practical reflection.

Interpreting

In this section I will make an interpretation of the first situation, based on what Carol has written and on what I can infer from the account. I realise that I am not the midwife in the action, so I will raise questions as a critical friend for Carol as necessary. Although there are two different accounts, the stories are about the communication complexities involved in managing the 'successful discharge' of mothers and babies from a postnatal unit.

Carol hoped for an effective discharge process of mothers and babies. I am unable to say how her hopes were related to her ideals of what constitutes 'good' practice, but I suspect that she considers that effective discharge processes are related to midwives knowing their role in the procedure and undertaking these responsibilities as part of their work activities. This role would involve a thorough knowledge of the process and the motivation and confidence to carry it out in reasonable time with minimal inconvenience to the mother, her family and the unit staff.

Only Carol can answer the questions about the sources in her life and work for her ideas and values for communicative aspects of her practice, and the ways she embodies them now in the way she communicates at work. However, as a critical friend, I noticed in the first situation that Carol did not mention speaking directly with the 'student midwife' involved, nor did she indicate that it was her intention to do so. Also, even though she had been given no notice of the impending discharge, Carol remedied the situation effectively, after a great deal of work, and she did not express her feelings directly.

In the first situation, Carol's communicative role was to use her knowledge and skills to manage a successful discharge of the mother and her twins. Although she achieved her communicative role in relation to the mother, the paperwork and the paediatrician, she may not have achieved it in relation to the student midwife. Carol could reflect on her intentions in this case, but as a critical friend, it seems to me that the student midwife is no more informed about how to fulfil the norms of managing a discharge process. This raises the issue of being direct in communication and letting people know how to improve their practice in future like cases.

Carol could ask herself how her interpretation of her role affected her relations with the people in the situation. She alone can make the connections between her role as she sees it and the way the situation unfolded. This is the point at which discoveries can be made that provide insights into favoured ways of being and working as a practitioner and the extent to which these behaviours can be reviewed and adapted.

When I considered the shared communication norms and expectations in this situation, I noticed that there were various people involved, including Carol, the student midwife, the mother and her babies and the paediatrician. All of the people in the situation would probably interpret their roles differently and have different expectations of the situation. For example, Carol knew her role in discharge procedures and managed it effectively. Carol had expectations that the student midwife knew the expectations of the role, but the story demonstrated that the student did not know the role, or that she was unwilling or unable to fulfil it. The mother acted in the role as the recipient of care and the paediatrican was a caregiver. It is possible that neither of these people was affected by the situation, as for them it went according to normal expectations, because Carol worked hard to fill in the gaps of knowledge and skill of the student midwife.

The expectation was that the student midwife would know and undertake the discharge procedure, and there were implicit sanctions in place to ensure the discharge procedure was effective. The student midwife did not appear to realise the effect of her inadequate communication in relation to this situation, but the sanction for ineffective midwifery care seems to be disapproval. I cannot name other forms of sanction, because Carol did not acknowledge her feelings in relation to this matter.

As I am unsure about the nature of the usual communicative norms and sanctions in Carol's practice, I cannot assume to know whether these patterns were altered in this situation. However, the answer to the question would assist Carol in understanding her role in this story.

Learning

In order to learn from this story, Carol could ask herself questions about her expectations of herself and of other people. This will show her the difference between her ideal and real practice and where the communicative action became confused or distorted. From these insights, Carol can learn from this situation and consider the kinds of adaptations, if any, that are possible in her work relationships. If Carol is able and willing to fit these new insights into her present ways of regarding communicative action in her work, she will have used the practical reflection process to increase her practice awareness and influence her own personal and professional growth and development.

SOME DISCUSSION ABOUT PRACTICAL REFLECTION

There are so many ways in which practical reflection can be helpful. For example, when you gain insights into what you usually think, say and do in certain situations in your work, you may begin to see that there are some aspects of your practice that have become habitual and relatively unexamined. Do you know the feeling of doing yet another day in the life of Nurse/Midwife ____ the ever-steady and ready worker? Can you be relied on to turn up at work, and to do the same kind of tasks day after day? After endless walking up and down corridors, getting in and out of work cars, entering more and more homes, units, wards and the like, are you still at it, labouring on relentlessly? Life and work can get tedious!

One way of fulfilling work commitments may be by coping on autopilot, so that you can handle routine tasks with minimal effort. In other words, you may be in a habit of facing work like a robot, to get tasks done well with minimal effort. Routine approaches can be useful in getting the work done, but they can also inhibit your spontaneous and appropriate human responses and communicative action. Routine practices may be robbing you of some of the purpose and pleasure you can derive from practice. Keep this idea in mind as you begin to reflect regularly.

When you did your first writing task in this book, you may have found that you have transposed certain childhood 'rules for living' into your adult work life as a practitioner. At this point, it is important to realise that some of your 'rules for living' may have become idealised. By this I mean that you may have come to see some of your rules as ultimate and unchangeable. There may be something so perfect about the content of the rules you have created for yourself that you feel you should always act in ways which are faithful to them and likely to fulfil their demands. This means that some of your favoured personal rules may be so unattainable that they may need another close look, in relation to what you think you should think, say and do in certain situations. There are some good reasons for doing this. Sometimes it is difficult to live up to your self-imposed ideals. For example, if you decided long ago that it is important to be loving and kind to everyone, the not-so-nice people you meet in your practice may cause you a great deal of internal turmoil and challenge your usual ways of communicating.

Nursing and midwifery have a way of levelling things out, so that what you idealise about today may be 'right in your face' tomorrow. The challenges in your practice can show you how hard it may be to 'walk your talk'. Practice has a way of bringing out some of the incongruencies between what you *say* you think, say and do and what you *actually* think, say and do. When practice is reflective, it can alert you to the differences between your espoused practice and your actual practice. Reflective practice will help you explore why the ideal and the real are not necessarily matched perfectly at all times, whether it is reasonable that they should be, and what can be done, if anything, about any mismatches.

It is possible to begin to imagine yourself as a person and practitioner, with qualities that are common to your private and work worlds. One of the things that you might like to consider as you pay attention to your work incidents is how you align your personal and work identities, and how these do and do not complement one another. You may be able to locate areas in which you are coming from your personal standpoints, or when you are coming from your work standpoints, or when these two perspectives have merged into an identity with no noticeable demarcation points. The reason for raising this issue is to alert you to the internal dialogue you can maintain with yourself and your critical friends about whether your personal and work worlds are separate, and whether this is desirable or reasonable. There are no right or wrong verdicts on this issue; rather, it is something you need to sort out yourself according to your specific set of personal characteristics and work circumstances. As this is such a large issue, it is worthy of your close and systematic reflection. The practical reflection process I have just described and applied can be very useful for this purpose, because it will assist you in understanding the relation of your personal and professional identities.

As you reflect on a regular basis, you will soon have many practice stories. To make sense of the connections between each story, review them carefully and locate your involvement in the stories by saying to yourself: 'It seems as if I think/feel . . .' If you take a different-coloured pen it will help if you actually write a note to yourself on the side of the entry or the creative representation you are using as a strategy for reflecting. This will mean that your journal or reflective portfolio of creative images will soon get a well-used look. By completing this sentence as often as you need to, you will find the things in practice that 'push your buttons,' and make you react each time they come up in some form or another. Most of us have our 'hobby horses' we get on and ride from time to time. Invariably, certain things never fail to surface, or to stir us up and make us uncomfortable in some ways. The chances are that you will find these themes in your reflection, even though initially your stories and representations appear to have little or no relation to one another. It may take some time before you can make these connections with ease; however, regular and frequent practice in reflection will ensure that you are able to move from the specific to the general in making sense of your work.

As you review your reflections, you may notice patterns of communication arising, such as the ways you react each time certain issues come up. For example, you may respond to a tone of voice, type of message, or other features of the person or persons communicating and the situation in which the interaction occurs.

When ideas arise as memories, they may need time to assimilate. Sometimes there is very little time between a memory and an insight, while at other times you may need longer to build on the initial ideas that arose at the time of the first insights. In other words, you may find that you will make more sense out of things after you have let the substance of them percolate for a while. As other ideas become connected, the insight deepens into something even more meaningful. So it is important now to take time during the process. You may only need to wait a few minutes between questions, or you may take hours or days. It is entirely up to you. However, it is also important not to delay so long that your flame of interest goes out. As with many things, timing is everything. You will know when you are ready to move on in the process and make sense of your reflections.

As you go through these reflective processes over the next few weeks or so, there may be times when you feel that you have made some discoveries about yourself as a person. If you have not been in the habit of thinking about yourself and the work you do, you may find that some of the reflective activities you are doing are somewhat confronting. It is OK to feel uncomfortable at times, because personal growth can emerge from this. You have probably heard the well-worn cliché: 'No pain, no gain'. This may apply to some extent, but it is also possible to grow through pleasure, so don't get hooked into thinking that if it's not hurting, it's not helping. In order to balance the number of confronting things with which you can deal at any one time, you should always remember that you are the one who chooses the depth of exploration and disclosure with which you feel most comfortable. This might mean that you look only at certain aspects of a situation, knowing there is more to come back to later. If you remember something which has enormous ramifications for you and you know you cannot do justice to it at a certain time in your life, you might even choose to leave it entirely until you are in a better frame of mind to deal with it. Don't forget this advice as you move on through the process. Enjoy the process. Practical reflection is a fun way of experiencing, interpreting and learning, so that you can grow and develop as a person and a professional.

SUMMARY

In this chapter I reviewed interpretive knowledge and practical interests in relation to practical reflection. I then guided you through a reflective exercise and presented and analysed some of Carol's stories about her midwifery experience. The chapter concluded with some discussion about practical reflection, in respect to the tendency nurses and midwives may have to try to be perfect, even if it is managed through habitual ways of doing tasks. I also discussed how to locate the recurring themes in your practice which can tell you about what 'pushes your buttons'. I suggested that practical reflection is an excellent means of experiencing, interpreting and learning to help you personally and professionally.

9

Emancipatory reflection

- Is this just another day at work, or is my 'good' day symptomatic of unexamined issues of power?
- What practices are so rcified in my work setting that they are not questioned?
- How can I improve my practice in spite of the constraints that work against me?

This chapter bring us to the third form of reflection. This will be helpful for you because it has the potential to answer these questions and more, and create some transformative action.

As I have reiterated throughout this book, you need not think of this form of reflection separately from the other forms, because in practice they merge into one another. However, it may be helpful for you to work through emancipatory reflection processes to show how they can assist you specifically in your work. By now, you will have noticed that there are many similarities in the forms of reflection and that the questions you ask yourself differ according to the focus of your practice issues. When you want to go beyond prediction provided by technical reflection, and description offered by practical reflection, it might be time to take a more critical view of your practice and the constraints within it. If you find that you are thwarted by the power relationships within your practice and work setting, you may need to adopt emancipatory reflective processes to bring about transformative action. In this chapter, I review some assumptions underlying emancipatory reflection before guiding you through the reflective processes and presenting and analysing one of Esther's stories to show you how nurses and midwives can transform their practice using these processes.

REVIEW OF PREVIOUS IDEAS

In Chapter 6 I explained that critical knowledge is derived from some key ideas in critical social science which have the potential to be emancipatory—that is, to have freeing possibilities. In particular, critical social science has the potential to free people from the oppression of their social and personal conditions. Critical theorising questions the status quo of various potentially repressive social contexts, to discover and expose the forces that maintain them for the advantages of particular people and regimes. This means that it looks at the way life is and asks how it might be different and better for the majority of people, not just for the privileged few who hold and use power. There are many key ideas in critical social science, but the ones I have included here for you to consider are the concepts of false consciousness, hegemony, reification, emancipation and empowerment. You will see that many of these ideas are related, and they describe the depth and scope of forces which can keep people controlled and subordinated.

False consciousness is the 'systematic ignorance that the members of . . . society have about themselves and their society' (Fay 1987: 27). *Hegemony* means the ascendancy or domination of one power over another, and it refers to the ways in which some social systems, and the people in them, give the impression that they are unassailable, and that the conditions they have produced are not only good, but also appropriate for the people over whom they have control. Nursing and midwifery settings have hegemonic influences operating within them and emancipatory reflection helps you to see where they are and how they create and maintain their power to work against you as a clinician.

Fay (1987: 92) explains that *reification* means 'making into a thing' and he defines it as 'taking what are essential activities and treating them as if they operated according to a given set of laws independently of the wishes of the social actors who engage in them'. These laws of social life are assigned a power of their own, thus becoming accepted and unquestioned as givens. As you can imagine, when practices become reified, they are immensely resistant to change because they are so deeply accepted that they can lie quietly in the background and thereby become relatively impervious to critique.

Emancipation means freedom, from your own and from other people's expectations and roles, and to adopt other self- and socially aware practices. *Empowerment* is the process of giving and accepting power, to liberate people from their oppressive circumstances. Emancipatory reflection alerts you to the possibilities of emancipation and gives you the means to empower yourself and others to have the courage to make a stand and bring about changes in the political system in which you work.

In summary, critical knowledge is potentially liberating for individuals and groups of people, when they realise that they may be living under misunderstandings about themselves and their social situations—misunderstandings which have been developed and held systematically. As people and practitioners, nurses and midwives are subject to oppressive social structures, which can be transformed through critical analysis and action. Emancipatory interest is rooted in power and it creates 'transformative action' which seeks to provide emancipation from forces which limit people's rational control of their lives. These forces are so influential and taken for granted that people have the strong impression such forces are beyond their control.

Emancipatory reflection involves human interaction, but it emphasises how people interpret themselves within their roles and social obligations. Emancipatory reflection leads to 'transformative action', which seeks to free nurses and midwives from taken-for-granted assumptions and oppressive forces which limit them and their practice. Emancipatory reflection provides you with a systematic means of critiquing the status quo in the power relationships in your workplace and it offers you raised awareness and a new sense of informed consciousness to bring about positive social and political change. Emancipatory reflection also offers you freedom from your own misguided and firmly held perceptions of yourself and your roles, to bring about change

196

for the better. The process of emancipatory reflection for change is *praxis*. Praxis in nursing and midwifery offers clinicians the means for change through collaborative processes that analyse and challenge existing forces and distortions brought about by dominating effects of power in human interaction.

APPLYING THE PROCESS

The work of Smyth (1986a) and Street (1991) is established in the area of emancipatory reflection. For many years now, nurses and midwives have been using this process with varying degrees of success, to construct, deconstruct, confront and reconstruct their practice. Please note, however, that authors such as Smyth and Street have not named this process 'emancipatory refection' as such, although it has a liberating intent.

Of all the forms of reflection, I consider that emancipatory reflection is the richest but riskiest, in terms of what it tries to do. It requires practitioners to make a deep, systematic and direct analysis of their work to locate the features which constrain effective practice. Given the hegemonic and reified conditions in work settings and relationships, this is no small task. Even so, the process has effects and rewards that can be so impressive as to change the habitual ways clinicians view themselves and go about their work.

Daily work incidents are the focus of emancipatory reflection and they are interactions in which you are active and central to what is happening. This means that practice incidents have within them all you need to construct, confront, deconstruct and reconstruct your practice. *Construction* of practice incidents allows you to describe, in words and other creative images and representations, a work scene played out previously, bringing to mind all of the aspects and constraints of the situation. *Deconstruction* involves asking analytical questions regarding the situation, which are aimed at locating and critiquing all the aspects of the situation. *Confrontation* occurs when you focus on your part in the scenario with the intention of seeing and describing it as clearly as possible. *Reconstruction* puts the scenario together again

197

with transformative strategies for managing changes in light of the new insights.

Important points to note

Although I endorse fully the potential of emancipatory reflection to bring about positive changes, I am very aware of the enormity of the task which faces any reflective practitioner who 'takes on the system'. In fact, I am so aware of the inherent dangers in the process that I have warned teachers of reflective practice that they should be careful about sending clinicians out prematurely and without ongoing support to fight 'big battles for small gains' (Taylor 1997). Even though I reflect on this issue often, and own up to my motherly need to protect novice reflective practitioners from the wilds of practice, I still feel that the process of emancipatory reflection is fraught with difficulties if it is applied in a 'gung ho' manner, without adequate support. With this in mind, I suggest that you find a colleague with whom to work collaboratively on your emacipatory reflection ventures. A critical friend may also be helpful, as he or she can act as another colleague, keeping you company on this journey of critical analysis (see Chapter 3).

Please note also that emancipatory reflection is only as helpful as the amount of effort you are willing to invest in making a thorough and systematic critique of the constraints within your practice. Emancipatory reflection will help you to analyse critically all of the features which have a bearing on your practice, whether they are personal, political, sociocultural, historical or economic. *Personal constraints* involve some unique features about nurses and midwives, into which you may or may not have insights. *Political constraints* are about work relationships and power struggles that happen day to day. The features of the workplace and how people define their entire ways of being together in that setting constitute *sociocultural constraints*. *Historical constraints* are those factors that have been inherited in a setting and which remain to cause difficulties. *Economic constraints* have to do with money, particularly a lack of it, in settings in which the health dollar is being made to stretch further and further. Nursing and midwifery practice can have some or all of these constraints, depending on particular work settings and the people interacting in them.

THE PROCESS OF EMANCIPATORY REFLECTION

As before, you are a central character in your practice stories, reflecting on your own practice as it relates to other people and determinants of the situation. When you have reflected on one scenario, you can go on to reflect on as many as you choose. Keep a record of all your reflections; they will be interesting to compare, because they track your reflective journey and they will show you your main issues and how you are working through them using reflective processes.

Choose an incident in which you were not entirely happy about the outcomes of your involvement—that is, you felt that you did not make a difference of a positive nature to someone in your care. The incident should also exemplify an imbalance of power and cooperation between people. The situation can involve as many people as you like, but you should be central in the activity. The following steps guide you through the reflective writing processes of construction, to describe the situation as fully as possible.

Constructing

In order to construct an incident in which you felt that you did not make a difference of a positive nature to someone in your care and there was an imbalance of power and cooperation between people, it might help to shut your eyes and take yourself back in your imagination to that time. You could also use other strategies to enhance your memory, such as those described in Chapter 3. When you have a clear image of the situation, write down, or represent creatively, a full description of the experience. If you respond to the following questions you will be able to build up a thick description of the event:

- What was happening?
- When was it happening?
- Where was it happening?

- What was the setting like, in terms of its smells, sounds and sights?
- Why was it happening?
- Who was involved?
- How were you involved?
- What were the outcomes of the situation?
- How did you feel honestly about the situation?

Now you need to review your construction of the situation.

- Is your description or creative representation as rich and full as possible?
- Does it capture the scene as faithfully as possible?

You might like to go back and elaborate further to ensure that you have described the experience as well as you possibly can. As you may have noticed already, a rich and full description at the outset provides more information on which to reflect.

Deconstructing

If you have been able to capture the context, you should have before you a fully descriptive scenario of the inter-actions and inherent power relations in an aspect of your practice. The reason I have described power relations as 'inherent' is that they will be there, but they may not be explicit at this point, especially as this story may not be able to capture all of the people's intentions and behaviours. Even if you use this process to describe a story in which events appear to go well, there may be implicit power plays operating. A critical view of practice helps you to see the power relations which bubble away, possibly just under the surface of what is apparent imme-diately. With this in mind, revisit your account or creative representation, and see what you can locate in terms of political motives and outcomes.

Identify your involvement in the scenario by looking at your part with the eyes of an interested observer standing back from the action. When you locate aspects of your contributions to the interaction, investigate your motives and actions by musing tentatively: 'It seems as if I act according to my belief that . . .' By completing this sentence as often as you need to, you will find the stimuli in practice that 'push your buttons' and make you react each time they come up in some form or another. The chances are that you will find these themes in your reflection, even though initially your practice stories appear to have little relation to one another.

Express yourself as clearly as you can, so that your observing self identifies, frankly and honestly, the person you have represented as yourself in the scenario. Write down or audiotape any observations you make, so that you can revisit them at a later time. Alternatively, you might like to write poetry or use some other creative means to respond to this part of the process. At this point, however, you need to be as clear in your mind as possible about what your musing means, so you need to make a note of your responses and interpret your creative reflections as they 'speak' to you presently.

Confronting

To become aware critically you need to remain vigilant and take a critical view of practice. Even when situations appear relatively positive, power interests may mediate them. To confront these power issues, you need to ask questions, such as:

- Where did the ideas I embody in my practice come from historically?
- How did I come to appropriate them?
- Why do I continue now to endorse them now in my work?
- Whose interests do they serve?
- What power relations are involved?
- How do these ideas influence my relationships with the people in my care? (Adapted from Smyth 1986a)

In being prepared to ask these questions, you are

making a critical analysis of your practice world. You will begin to see that, even though you are often at the centre of your world, you are certainly not the only determinant of the situation. The world in which you exist and act is influenced by historical, sociocultural, economic and political determinants, which to greater and lesser extents constrain the ways in which you are free to interpret and act in your world in any given moment. The realisation that you are 'not alone' in your practice can free you from bitter self-recriminations and raise the possibilities of new awareness. At some stage it may also be possible to transform the repressive conditions which cause you to act in certain ways.

Reconstructing

Reconstructing puts the scenario together again with transformative strategies for managing changes in light of the new insights. Given that you have been able to follow the process of systematic inquiry outlined so far, by now you may have realised that there may be contradictions in what you say you think, *say* and do, and what you *actually* think, say and do. You may have also realised that what you do is also affected by historical, sociocultural, economic and political determinants of the setting in which you work, which cause you to act in certain ways in your practice world.

The only remaining step in the process of emancipatory reflection, then, is to free yourself to the possibilities of using your raised awareness in reconstructing your world. There may be a lot of space between raised awareness and change, but if you do not allow yourself to imagine the possibilities of transformation, then nothing will be possible. If you dare to imagine and to plan to act in ways that are capable of transforming your world, then you will have attempted to break out of the taken-for-granted assumptions which maintain the status quo and serve the interests of the people who are in positions of domination, whomever they may be in your particular reality.

The final question to be posed is:

- In the light of what I have discovered, how might I work differently?

As you imagine some different ways of acting, don't forget that you are not alone in your work setting. Consider how historical, sociocultural, economic and political determinants might play a part in the way you are able to work. Begin to imagine or make some adjustments to some of the situational constraints as part of your plan of action for change.

AN EXAMPLE OF EMANCIPATORY REFLECTION

In this section I present, verbatim, Esther's story about caring for a critically ill newly birthed young woman before transfer to a larger hospital. As before, I have not adjusted the story for grammar, expression or any other criterion, so that you can see the value of writing according to your own style. Esther writes descriptively, so it gives her a lot of information with which to work. In this story, she refers to a previous situation, which has been included in Chapter 2 of this book, to exemplify the kinds of issues midwives face in their practice. You might like to go back and review Esther's other story, as it reiterates the frustration she expresses here about her perceptions of inadequate medical support in caring for women during labour and delivery.

A woman was admitted for an elective induction of labour at 38 weeks' gestation. She was exceptionally obese and hypertensive. She had obvious ankle oedema. On examination, her Bishop's score was unfavourable for artificially rupturing her membranes. I had looked after this woman when a similar situation had arisen in her previous pregnancy, and she was transferred to the Base Hospital for intrapartum care. In that incident, my intervention regarding the inappropriateness of her birthing at our hospital, which is only accredited for low-risk, normal deliveries, was not appreciated. However, she was transferred to specialist, obstetric care, which she needed, and deserved!

Now the same nightmare scenario was repeating itself! I was really pissed off, as whoever (and I knew who) had completed her antenatal booking had not either recognised her at-risk condition, or done anything about it, i.e. phoned the GP/obs or discussed the situation with the hospital manager. Therefore, this woman had presented inappropriately again!

Her blood pressure was sky high and she had protein in her urine. As usual, it was after hours. I phoned the nurse manager II. She empathised but wouldn't intervene. She told me to phone the hospital manager. I did, explained the situation and was told that the GP/obs was under no circumstances to do an ARM. When the GP arrived, he was to phone the hospital manager.

The GP arrived, ignored the request to phone the hospital manager and went to see the woman. He disagreed with our findings of hypertension. He examined her vaginally and lo, her membranes ruptured! Quite a coincidence—however, the liquor was heavily meconium stained, and the fetal heart rate, extremely difficult to locate because of her obesity, became erratic, bradycardia, tachycardia and some Type II dips.

By this stage, the night duty staff had come on, so a new midwife was left with the fiasco. The subsequent story was one of transfer to the Base Hospital, and emergency Caesarean. Another case study to the hospital manager, another story of inappropriate medical care and nothing done to change the situation! The GP in question continues to be reaccredited for obstetrics despite not meeting the recommended criteria of births/triennium!! We all wondered the reason that this particular woman continues to choose this GP for her obstetric care!

Collusive behaviour between some midwives, inept GPs and gutless management ensures that the status quo remains, inept, dangerous practice continues and obstetric/midwifery care is sometimes poor, depending on the midwife and GP involved.

Deconstructing these two incidents is not difficult as, unfortunately, they happen quite frequently when the two GPs cited are involved. The interests served are definitely those of maintaining the status quo, i.e. medically dominated birthing. The power relations are that of oppression—of birthing women and midwives on the one hand—and domination by general practitioners. Women are given very little choice or information, therefore informed decision-making re birthing is limited.

My relationship with the women in my care while practising midwifery is definitely influenced by the power relations. There continues to be a dilemma where my strong belief in advocacy is challenged by both the GPs (the two already cited, in particular) and in a more insidious way, by some midwives. Evidence-based practice is the norm for very few, and therefore, best practice outcomes are frustratingly difficult to achieve. Paternalistic, medically dominated intrapartum care suits some women, however, and this is where my relationships are most difficult, as some women do choose not to be an active participant in birthing, and just want it over and done with! Encountering these women is a good learning experience, though, as my tolerance and acceptance really needs practice then!

After reassuring myself that these women truly aren't interested in participating actively in birthing from informed choice rather than ignorance, i.e. limited or no information from GP, antenatal classes, etc. and offering lots of different options and information on possible outcomes connected to choices, I will support the women in my care to the utmost of my ability. However, if their choices are ones which I believe will adversely affect them or their babies, I will advocate strongly for different strategies/interventions, despite their GP's opinion.

The themes within the stories so far are those which demonstrate oppressive/dominant behaviours and relationships, collusive and acquiescent behaviours and poor practice, culminating in less than optimal outcomes for mother and baby. These themes will always push my buttons while they exist in midwifery, and I will continue to act to prevent them occurring.

Reconstruction of these events in terms of—in light of what I have discovered, how might I work differently? gives rise to the question, what can I do differently to change obsolete, ineffective and potentially dangerous practice—both obstetric and midwifery? I need to be more creative in achieving change. Some ways which may help—give this journal to my hospital manager and others to read, so that they may understand what is happening. The hospital manager is newly appointed and may be *more willing to advocated better maternity care rather than maintenance of amenable relationships with paternalistic GPs. Continue with proactivity— initiate discussion of unfavourable outcomes—use case studies as inservice so that it is seen as a learning experience and an opportunity to improve care. Push for reexamination of GP/obs and anaes- thetist accreditation—argue the lack of cost effective practice when GPs are participating in three to four births a year and still being allocated a Rural Incentive grant (worth about $8000) to help with insurance—I've already given some figures to the Health Service Area DON and I will follow up what she had done about it. Also discuss this with the hospital manager—he's not a midwife and has limited understanding of the issues involved, I surmise.*

APPLYING AN EMANCIPATORY REFLECTION PROCESS

As you can see from Esther's story, she has already applied the emancipatory process to construct, deconstruct, confront and reconstruct her practice. Even so, it might be useful to revisit the story. Acting in the role of critical friend, I will provide some commentary on the situation and let you know about subsequent thoughts Esther has had on this and other practice occasions which required her to be critically aware and proactive.

Constructing

Esther constructed the scene of the incident well, especially regarding the imbalance of power and cooperation between herself, the other midwives and the doctor involved. She described clearly what was happening, when, where and why. Although Esther did not describe the setting in terms of its smells, sounds and sights, she constructed the scene carefully in terms of who was involved, how she was involved and the outcomes of the situation. We are also left in no doubt as to how Esther felt about the situation.

Deconstructing

When Esther revisited the story to see what she could locate in terms of political motives and outcomes, she had plenty of justification for feeling that the woman was mismanaged by the midwife who booked her in as low risk, and the doctor who she felt acted inappropriately in giving medical care. In doing this, however, she jumped quickly to conclusions, without engaging in a more tentative process. For example, Esther wrote: 'Collusive behaviour between some midwives, inept GPs and gutless management ensures that the status quo remains, inept, dangerous practice continues and obstetric/midwifery care is sometimes poor, depending on the midwife and GP involved.' Whereas this judgment may or may not have some 'truth' and merit, it is important at this point for Esther to identify her involvement in the scenario, by looking at her part with the eyes of an interested observer standing back from the action.

Esther could make explorations tentatively, using the detector statement of: 'It seems as if I intend/act according to my belief that . . .' By completing this sentence as often as she needs to, she could find the basis for the events in practice that 'push her buttons' and make her react each time they come up in some form or another. For example, it seems as if Esther had standards of care, which may or may not have been met by midwives and doctors, which she applied to management situations. Only Esther can apply this tentative exploration of herself in other respects. For instance, she may see that it seems as if she has certain unexamined ideas about how she views 'good' practice, or that her frustration at incompetence may be connected to a deeply personal part of her life. I raise these ideas purely as conjecture.

Confronting

To become more aware critically, Esther could confront these and other power issues by asking herself where the ideas she embodies in her practice came from historically, how she came to appropriate them, and why she continues to endorse them now in her work. Although Esther came close to answering these questions, she veered off and did not quite address them. For example, she concluded:

> The interests served are definitely those of maintaining the status quo, i.e. medically dominated birthing. The power relations are that of oppression—of birthing women and midwives on the one hand—and domination by general practitioners. Women are given very little choice or information, therefore informed decision making re birthing is limited.
>
> My relationship with the women in my care while practising midwifery is definitely influenced by the power relations. There continues to be a dilemma where my strong belief in advocacy is challenged by both the GPs (the two already cited, in particular) and in a more insidious way, by some midwives . . .

In response to what I thought might be a tendency to reach conclusions rapidly, during a phone call one day in which Esther was describing her experience of becoming a reflective practitioner, I asked her to put herself into the picture. It seemed to me that in her quest to name the problem and put things right, Esther did not involve herself, but she seemed to draw conclusions about other people's motives and behaviour. Esther said she would think about what I said and I received the following response when she submitted her stories for inclusion in this book.

A phone call from Bev to check whether I still wanted to be involved with her project. I got the impression that she was pleased that I had done so much.

I read Bev one of my practice incidents and the accompanying deconstruction and reconstruction to her, and she provided comment, empathy and feedback. She was really pleased with what I've done. However, she did note the lack of emotional content, and requested some personal/emotional/feeling additions to my narration.

So . . . here goes. When Bev commented on my lack of emotionality, and asked for feelings to be included, my voice became really chokey, and I almost started crying.

I know that I keep a lot of emotional stuff damped down regarding my nursing and midwifery practice and the culture within which I work, because if I didn't, I'd either be constantly angry, or a blubbering mess, or both!

The injustices within midwifery (and nursing—I can speak for both, working in the multi-skilled environment of a small rural hospital!) are sometimes too much to bear. I sometimes wonder whether, if I didn't love my locality so much, and didn't have a family content and happy here, whether I'd stay. Certainly, when I first arrived from Sydney I was totally shocked by the nepotistic, medically dominated, conservative, class ridden structures within the Health Service. That opinion hasn't changed much.

However, given my personal situation, and the fact that my spiritual beliefs are interwoven with socialist beliefs which recognise the right of every sentient being to equal access to health care and education of comparative worth/value, I won't/can't give up. I will whittle away the injustices for clients and staff little by little. I couldn't live with integrity if I didn't.

So, I endeavour to see the good in everyone, thank those who aggravate or anger me for the ability to practise compassion (what a challenge) and ensure my levels of courage and hope remain high by networking with like-minded colleagues.

Oh, but I feel sooooo alone sometimes. I had two soul mates in midwifery at work for a short couple of months. They couldn't/wouldn't handle the injustice, oppression, domination, nepotism, poor practice, etc., etc., and moved on. I don't blame them, but I'll miss their support. My husband supports me and sustains me, as do friends and colleagues in similar situations in other hospitals.

Sometimes I despair that the medically dominated culture in rural midwifery will ever change. However, doing things like participating in this project helps me to clarify my thoughts and feelings, and consequently, motivates me to continue.

I will share this journal with my hospital manager and my area DON. I don't think that they will like what they read. However, it may be a way to put them in the skin of a midwife who is really trying to practise with integrity, courage and vision. Maybe, just maybe, it may be a jumping off point for change!!!!

PLEASE . . .

I must also say that I am definitely not perfect in either my attitudes or my practice. I tend to be judgmental regarding others who are judgmental! So the process of lifelong reflection continues and trying to learn/improve.

Writing this journal has really given me a push to share my experiences/feelings regarding mid-wifery with those who may be able to help me to achieve needed change. I have felt at a bit of a stalemate, as other colleagues do not have the passion I have to ensure improved maternity care becomes a reality. By passing this journal on to others who are actually in a position to initiate change, it will at least give them an insight into one midwife's professional life.

From her writing, we can see how Esther responded to the questions about interests and power relations, and how these issues influenced her relationships with the people in her care. Esther has begun to make a critical analysis of her practice world, and to recognise that it is influenced by historical, sociocultural, economic and political determinants.

Reconstructing

In reconstructing the scenario, Esther suggested some transformative strategies for managing changes in light of the her new insights. For example, she referred to sharing her journal to let people see how she was reflecting on her practice issues. When she asked herself how she might work differently in the light of what she had discovered, she reviewed some of the constraints. She wrote:

What can I do differently to change obsolete, ineffective and potentially dangerous practice—both obstetric and midwifery? I need to be more creative in achieving change. Some ways which may help—give this journal to my hospital manager and others to read, so that they may understand what is happening. The hospital manager is newly appointed and may be more willing to advocate better maternity care rather than maintenance of amenable relationships with paternalistic GPs. Continue with proactivity— initiate discussion of unfavourable outcomes—use case studies as inservice so that it is seen as a learning experience and an opportunity to improve care. Push for reexamination of GP/obs and anaesthetist accreditation—argue the lack of cost effective practice when GPs are participating in three to four births a year and still being allocated a Rural Incentive grant (worth about $8000) to help with insurance—I've already given some figures to the Health Service Area DON and I will follow-up what she

> *had done about it. Also discuss this with the hospital manager—he's not a midwife and has limited understanding of the issues involved, I surmise.*

As part of the process of working with the nurses and midwives, whose stories feature in this book, I sent the typed transcript of their writing, so that they could check it for errors and provide additions and areas to be excluded. Esther wrote this message to me in pen on the transcript I sent her.

> *Bev,*
> *I have started to initiate the changes suggested in the journal. I am organising relevant inservice for midwives and promoting evidence based practice to empower midwives to explore alternative options. My EO/DON was given a copy of the journal, and since then, he has been very supportive of working toward improving/enhancing maternity care, and although not a midwife himself, has come up with some innovative strategies to ensure that all midwives continue their education. I am giving increased time to our local midwives group and we hope to have a shared care maternity model commencing in the not too distant future.*
> *The midwives in the Health Service are also enthusiastic for me to do a horizontal violence/oppression workshop at a seminar next year, and that may hopefully tackle issues of medical dominance and raise midwives' consciousness.*
> *So, proactivity rules, and things look reasonably positive. Apart from this addendum, the transcript is fine, barring some typos.*

I look forward to a copy of the finished product, if that is possible.
Regards,
Esther

Esther was prepared to use the emancipatory reflection process to look carefully at her practice and to make some changes within it. You may have realised by now that this kind of process takes energy, time and courage, but it is not too difficult and it can be successful in measured amounts over time. Because this process drives at the very core of what keeps practice unquestioned and unchanged, it represents risky behaviour to use intentionally a process which is geared towards uptipping hegemony and all of the influences operating in power relationships in practice. Even so, how thrilling to try! Esther's story shows you what is possible if you approach practice issues carefully and systematically. It is possible to create change strategies and for them to have an influence on the ways practice happens in health care settings.

DISCUSSION ABOUT EMANCIPATORY REFLECTION

If you are working through this book sequentially, by now you are probably well on the way to making sense out of your practice, by focusing on your experiences of it. Even though you may be locating rewarding aspects of your practice, you may also be uncovering values, beliefs and behaviours which are important. If you take a closer look at these events, you may start to see that your responses take on certain features in situations you judge as positive or negative. It may transpire that you realise that you begin to feel uncomfortable in situations in which positive features are missing. It might be a valuable exercise to ask yourself why.

For example, you may find that that you tend to feel most comfortable about work situations that are predictable, where there are no uncertainties or unexpected outcomes. Similarly, you may feel good about situations in which it is shown that you have acted correctly or you were congratulated for work well done. While these examples are positive, they can also shed some light on the conditions you choose for yourself which make you feel most comfortable at work. In other words, these examples might also tell you that you are a practitioner who needs to be in control of situations. To what extent does your need for control limit other people's freedom?

If you always need to feel you have acted correctly, are there ways in which you have made yourself feel the need to be 'Super Nurse', or 'Super Midwife', who is always correct, even on relative human issues, which do not necessarily have right or wrong outcomes? If you have a strong need to be congratulated for work well done, you might like to consider why. Does this mean that you do not have your own mechanisms for self-appreciation? To what extent do you rely on other people for your sense of self-worth? Or, it is possible that you crave appreciation because you work in a culture which does not acknowledge work well done? These examples are meant to be representative of the kinds of questions you might ask yourself even when your practice seems to be going positively. The questions are not posed to raise self-doubt, but to question some taken-for-granted assumptions you might be making about yourself, your work setting and the way you work. They rest on an assumption that you can always improve the way you are and work, and that you can question the constraints in your work context, so that you practise more effectively.

As I mentioned previously, emancipatory reflection will help you to see that, even though you are often at the centre of your practice world, you are certainly not the only reason why it might be judged positive or negative. Even though some personal constraints may be operative, political, sociocultural, historical and economic constraints may also be in play. For example, nurses and midwives working in hospitals may find that they are thwarted in their practice to some extent by the political nature of the hierarchical relationships between themselves and some doctors. They may also be working under conditions in which they are short staffed, with little or no hope of relief. The social and cultural aspects of working in a setting may include expectations that they will fetch, carry and clean up afterwards for doctors. Nurses and midwives may tend to perpetuate these routines because they have been entrenched historically and for other reasons of which they may need to become aware. You might even say: 'We do it like this, because it has always been this way!'

It is a liberating thought to realise that the personal and work worlds in which you exist and act are influenced by historical, sociocultural, economic and political determinants, which to greater and lesser extents constrain the ways in which you are free to interpret and act in your situation at any given moment. The realisation that you are 'not alone' in your practice can free you from bitter self-recriminations that it was your fault that events went 'wrong'. Even though your training and education as a nurse or midwife may have encouraged you to think that you were singularly responsible for the good health of the entire Western world, this is simply not so. Knowing that you do not act in a vacuum, and that you act and are acted upon in certain ways, can raise the possibilities of new awareness. First, it can absolve you from the guilt of not being a perfect nurse or midwife. Second, this awareness may be the basis of the transformation of your repressive conditions.

Looking at your own practice in order to raise your awareness about your own values and action also encourages you to shift your focus outwards towards the situation in which you work and how you interact within that context. When you ask the question: 'What or whose interests are being served?' you shift the focus from yourself alone to the social and political issues in which you are immersed. Emancipatory reflection, therefore, is directed towards freeing interests. In other words, emancipatory reflection is able to free you to other possibilities, however limited or grand they may be.

Be as honest with yourself as you can be. Explore as many ideas as come to mind, so that you can leave yourself open to multiple possibilities. Be sure that you do not foreclose on your insights too early. In other words, don't jump to rapid conclusions and shut off the possibilities of other explanations. A way of managing this might be to write in a tentative fashion. For example: 'It seems that the ideas I live out now come from many sources. Some of them might be . . .' As you make these statements, continue to own your part in the analysis, by referring to yourself in the first person (I, my, me, mine). At the same time, be sure to cast your gaze wider than the personal factors at play. Remember to examine all of the other determinants which may be constraining the situation.

Granted, there is a lot of space between raised awareness and change, but if you do allow yourself to imagine the possibilities of transformation, then something will be possible. If you dare, you can imagine, plan and act in ways that are capable of transforming your world. You can attempt to break out of the taken-for-granted assumptions which maintain the status quo in which you work. These forces serve the interests of the people who are in positions of domination, whoever they may be in your particular reality.

Don't forget, though, that the initial changes may be very small, and some of them may even seem insignificant. You will not necessarily change overnight the entire system or the way you work as an individual. Reaching too far too soon may lead to disappointment, so take the process slowly, watching for changes along the way, and adding them to your repertoire of experiences as a practitioner.

SUMMARY

This chapter presented the third form of reflection, which has the potential to answer questions about power relationships and create some transformative action in your work. I suggested that when you want to go beyond prediction provided by technical reflection and description offered by practical reflection, that it might be time to take a more critical view of your practice using emancipatory reflection. To that end, I reviewed some assumptions underlying emancipatory reflection, before I guided you through the reflective processes. Esther shared her practice story and I analysed it as a critical friend, to show you how nurses and midwives can transform their practice using emancipatory reflection. I hope you can apply the processes in this chapter and that you enjoy the practice changes they bring about.

10

Experiences and reflections

I have found that nurses and midwives love to tell and hear stories so, with this in mind, in this chapter I provide you with opportunities to read more practice stories from Esther, Michael and Carol. Through sharing their stories with you, these clinicians offer you a means of improving your reflective skills and knowledge. You can analyse their stories to locate their practice approaches, issues and themes, and provide your commentary to them as a critical friend; in so doing, you will be able to learn from their experience. You can also read the comments and questions I make to them in the role of their critical friend. Many of the issues raised here 'cut very close to the bone' and may be highly contentious for some readers. Nursing and midwifery practice can be confronting and I make no apologies for the gut-wrenching realities in these stories. The inclusion of these stories in this book bears testimony to the courage of practitioners in being willing to face their fears and frustrations and I honour that courage with my frank and direct commentary.

SHARING STORIES

The stories which follow appear as they were written by Esther, Michael and Carol. You will notice that each clinician has a different writing style and he or she has made a particular interpretation of how to write for reflection. I am not putting these stories up as excellent examples of how to write reflectively, even though each person has made a strong commitment towards doing well. These stories are included to show you how some clinicians have written and to demonstrate that any kind of writing can be used as a basis for reflection. Even though I have emphasised the need to be as descriptive as possible, not everyone starts out or catches on to writing in this way. So, rather than write nothing—and therefore fail to reflect—I want you to be encouraged by the efforts of these three clinicians and try to write reflectively also.

As you read these stories, I would like you to practise reading carefully for issues and ways in which you could raise questions and suggestions to assist the clinician. At the end of each set of stories, I will raise certain areas on which you can focus, to hone your skills in being a critical friend, while you develop your knowledge and skills about being a reflective practitioner.

As I have emphasised before, the clinicians' accounts are as they wrote them. I have left the writing as it is purposefully, so that you can read the accounts as they have been written, to show you that there is nothing difficult or intimidating about writing for reflection.

Esther's stories

A story about a sick baby

It was a morning shift and I had just taken over from the night duty midwife. A woman had just delivered and was postnatally well. However, the baby had had a tachypnoea and grunting respirations since birth, possibly due to aspirating liquor as the membranes had not ruptured until the babe was being born. The night duty midwife had put the baby in a humidicrib for observation, although the babe's parents objected to this. They had finally been persuaded that it was in the baby's

219

interests. The GP/obs had left in a rush, stating that he had a birthday party to organise, that he wasn't worried about the baby and that if we needed to discuss the babe's condition with anyone, to phone Dr B.

With this information in my head, I went to check the babe. He was indeed respiratorily distressed. I set up the pulse oximetry machine and found that the babe's sats were unacceptably low. I then organised some oxygen to be fed into the crib and went to reread the notes. I noted that the GP had written that he suspected that the baby had 'a wet lung'. He had not mentioned this to anyone else. I rang the GP, Dr B, who was supposed to be covering and was told that he was actually out of town, and therefore, could not have been contacted. I then asked the GP on-call at our hospital to check the babe for me. He did, and concurred with my findings. However, due to the parent's ambivalence/ denial of the babe's condition, he proposed to review the babe in one hour. I kept a close eye on the babe, and before the hour was up, got the on-call GP in for a review—the babe's condition was deteriorating and I had managed to explain to the parents just what we were concerned about. They had been relying on the first GP's assessment that there was 'nothing to be concerned about'.

The on-call GP phoned our Base Hospital, spoke to a paediatrician, and we transferred the babe. He was subsequently diagnosed with aspiration pneumonia and commenced on IV antibiotics.

Deconstructing this incident, the GP's interests are clearly being served. The power relations were such that the GP/obs had not considered it necessary to communicate effectively regarding the baby's condition—who knows why? However, his ambivalence and ineffective communication meant that I both needed to advocate on the baby's behalf, and clarify the situation to parents who could not comprehend the gravity of the situation. It was not until I requested a second GP to assess the babe that the parents began to understand. They assumed that the first GP knew best ?because he was a doctor and I was a midwife or ?because he is a male and I am a female. Who knows—it wasted precious time!

Reconstruction means looking at how I might work differently. In that situation, I believe that my practice was effective and professional and if I had to do anything differently, it would be to have discussed the situation with the GP/obs later (which I didn't), as it seems to me that his practice was unaccountable, and that he may well have benefited by reflecting on the outcome of his ambivalence.

A critical friend's commentary and questions

In this story I detected Esther's concern about a sick baby and her frustration about lack of medical communication and care. The situation demanded Esther's quick thinking, assessment and action and the favourable outcome in correcting the baby's condition was attributable directly to her expert practice.

I offer these questions to Esther as a critical friend:

- What other assumptions are possible in explaining the parents' inability 'to comprehend the gravity of the situation'?
- What are the possible reasons for not discussing the situation after the event with the GP?

A story about lying down for labour

Another incident, fairly brief, but significant in terms of client (birthing) outcomes.

Morning shift—a primip in 2nd stage of labour—very tired and not pushing effectively, according to night duty midwife. I walked in to the birthing room with the midwife finishing her shift, and found the woman lying flat on her back, pushing ineffectively. The night duty midwife left quickly. After quickly assessing the woman, I suggested that her efforts may be more effective if she got up and either stood, or squatted. She did, and the baby was born reasonably soon afterwards. I was angry that this woman had been denied appropriate guidance and support which would have shortened her labour.

Deconstruction—I don't honestly know whose interests were being served in this incident. Certainly not the birthing woman's! I suppose that also applies to the power relations. I believe that it was more lack of education (both midwife and client) that lead to the situation, and that is certainly related to historical, sociocultural, economic and political determinants driven by medically dominated maternity care which the client and the night duty midwife had obviously accepted as the norm. So, indirectly, even though the GP wasn't present, it was that medical dominance which influenced the incident.

Reconstruction—Once again, I was able to turn things around for the client, which I find I do, not often, but on occasion, depending on the care and practice of the previous midwife (and continuing education in midwifery!)

In retrospect, I needed to speak to the midwife. I didn't, because of shifts, days off, etc., however, I regret that I didn't.

Writing about this incident has really energised me to talk to my hospital manager regarding midwifery continuing education, as very few of the midwives here practise effectively, utilising evidence-based research, etc. Its much easier to acquiesce to the medical model of women lying flat on their backs to birth. So, I need to ensure that midwifery is given a much higher profile here.

A critical friend's commentary and questions

In this story, Esther was angry that a birthing woman had been left on her back to deliver. Although the midwife going off duty was directly responsible, Esther concluded that the fault really resided with doctors, who required a back lying position for easier biomedical management during delivery.

I offer these questions to Esther as a critical friend:

- You have concluded that medical dominance influenced this incident, yet it is another example of you coming in to remedy a clinical situation, in this case caused directly by another midwife. When you review this story and compare it with others shared with us here, what does it tell you about yourself, in terms of your tendency to fix situations? Can you identify ways in which your rules for living you described previously have influenced your tendency to want to fix situations?
- How can you help other people to learn from your intervention? I am alluding here to your tendency to fix problems without going directly to the person involved, in this case, the night shift midwife.

When you look over these two stories offered by Esther, read carefully to see if you can locate issues and themes that seem to keep on coming up for her. Imagine that you are acting as Esther's critical friend and consider ways in which you could raise these issues and themes with her so that she is best able to make sense of them for herself. It might help you to turn to Chapter 4 to review Esther's description of childhood influences on her life and the section on how to be a critical friend.

Michael's stories

A story about intravenous site pain

Another frustrating situation I found myself in recently is also on a night shift. Mr A was one week post-op from a spinal fusion with an anterior approach. His post-op recovery had been quite eventful with a bowel obstruction and DVT post-op. Mr A was on a heparin IV to anticoagulate him. An anxious man pre-operatively, Mr A was very aware of every move and every detail of care provided.

During the day Mr A had complained of pain radiating up the arm where the heparin IV was sited. The IV had been resited and now Mr A stated that he had instant relief. The physician looking after Mr A had made a comment to nursing staff about the nature of pain not being genuine as a result of this claim. The physician believed that the patient was possibly hyper-sensitive due to the excessive amounts of pethidine the patient was receiving. A strong possibility given it had been given second hourly for one week. In the early hours of the morning Mr A began complaining of severe pain radiating up the arm from the IV site. In the absence of any differing analgesic orders I gave the patient pethidine which had little effect on the pain.

When the pain was reaching the stage when the pain was unbearable I phoned the physician at home (about 1.30am). When I explained the pain and how pethidine had not relieved the pain the physician began to get annoyed that I had given pethidine as he believed this was the source of the problem as the 'heparin IV does not cause pain'. I explained that I would be happy to give something else for pain if the doctor would prescribe it. To this the doctor answered that Heparin does not cause pain and that this was all in the patient's mind and that he would not prescribe anything for the pain. (Another physician to strike from the list!)

In Melbourne there was a well known oncologist Walter Moon who has been quoted in pain management lectures around Melbourne as saying that pain = suffering and pain is whatever the person suffering describes it as—a great shame Dr L had never attended one of these lectures. I however was left to try and manage a patient crying with pain in the middle of the night. I went back to the patient and tried to rationalise what the prick of a doctor had told me, that is, it was unlikely the heparin is the cause of the pain and as such I was unable to cease the infusion. I also told him that as Dr L had believed pethidine to be the cause of the problem I would manage his pain as best I could with hot packs and oral analgesia. This lasted for one hour before the patient was threatening to pull the IV out. I rang Dr L again, as usual the second call gets them listening as they realise they may not get to sleep well. This time the doctor ordered Largactil (great I think as this can enhance the effect of analgesia). Then comes the crunch—5mg orally—

barely enough to help a child much less an adult male with chronic pain management problems. I argue the dose with the doctor, who does not give at all. Realising I am getting nowhere I terminate the call.

At this point the woman I am working with states that we'll have to allow for spillage with the Largactil syrup. Not usually being one to do this I agree and the patient settles eventually another hour later. When I come on duty the next night the patient is a different person—the IV remains in and causing no pain. The patient has had no further pethidine and is a different person. Dr L was right (about the pethidine) and I don't begrudge him that it was a tough call. What I am frustrated with is that this guy has got away with making subjective statements about a patient's pain or refused to treat the pain. I ask the Unit Manager to pull the Medical Director (a pain management specialist) aside and inform him during the day, I know well that nothing will be done but hope that some day a patient will challenge this doctor or his attitude.

A critical friend's commentary and questions

In this story I detected a number of issues, which overlapped one another. For example, Michael was keen to relieve Mr A's pain and he used the only drug ordered at the time, pethidine, even though the physician suspected that the patient was hypersensitive to pain. Within this issue was Michael's annoyance about the physician making subjective comments about the patient's estimation of his pain and the doctor's statement about intravenous heparin not causing pain. There was also a conflict with the doctor about obtaining an order for a drug to relieve the patient's pain, Michael's displeasure at the amount of Largactil allowed, and the very serious issue of

Michael intentionally giving more drug than ordered by allowing 'for spillage'.

I offer these questions to Michael as a critical friend:

- What are the issues here and how are they related to one another?
- Why were you willing to disregard the *Poisons Act* and give more than the ordered dose of a drug to this patient?
- You made the comment: 'Not usually being one to do this … (go against a drug order)'. What nursing practice issues are so important for you that you would risk subverting the system for them? Why?

A story about knowing when it is time to die

Betty E was a woman in her 70s, two days post-knee replacement when I nursed her in HOU on a Saturday night. I arrived on duty on a cold wintry night to find the door to HOU wide open and a fan going to feed Betty's hunger for air. A long history of bilateral mastectomy, COAD, smoker—50 years, TKR meant it was no surprise to the physician involved in Betty's case that she was like this and when they met as they had late Saturday evening there would be a bit of banter rather than anything constructive come of his visits.

After an hour or two of nursing Betty I knew that at some stage in the near future Betty would have a respiratory arrest. I guess it was clinical knowledge combined with intuition that made me arrive at this. It was confirmed when Betty told me she wouldn't make it through this one.

I don't try to stop people from talking like this at any stage as it is so important to know what the patients are thinking so I answered with my typical answer that she had just been through some major surgery and was she prepared to give in so easily? Betty pointed to her chest where the

---

mastectomies had been performed and informed me that she had done her share of fighting. I couldn't argue that at all.

I watched Betty overnight with a pulse of 102, ST regular as you like. Resp rate between 18–22, O$_2$ saturation—97%, waiting for something that would indicate what I thought was inevitable, whilst at the same time frustrated by the private system that I work in where you don't have access to medical staff when you have a significant event overnight, so I was not able to ring the physician and say what I thought would happen. Instead, I would have to wait until something indicated in Betty's medical condition.

I went off duty at 0730 and at 0930 Betty had a respiratory arrest in the presence of medical staff. Intubation was difficult and as a consequence, Betty was ventilated for 48 hours then the ventilator turned off due to brain death. She died four hours later.

If you spend some time analysing Michael's stories, you will see that he has certain practice approaches and similar issues and themes surface from time to time. I was able to contact Michael for discussion during the time he was writing some of his practice stories for this book. I mentioned to him that there seemed to be issues about acknowledgement arising in many of his stories. This is what he wrote in reply to my suggestion.

Discussions with a critical friend

I talked the first part of my journal over with Bev. She asks me what I see as the common theme (I don't as yet). The thing I find satisfying is when I feel I am a part of the healing process. Bev sees this as maybe wanting acknowledgement or acceptance. This blows me away as I recall the common themes from my childhood—all women as key people, the issue of acceptance, my struggle for acceptance rather than tolerance from my family.

I guess the relationship I have with patients is a very comfortable one because issues of sexuality are irrelevant. When you're caring for a patient in a professional manner the patient does not care about your sexuality. It certainly has never been an issue for me, but I guess I don't stand out as being gay and don't 'flaunt' my sexuality. Flaunt is a really ugly word to use when describing sexuality but it is the early hours of the morning and I am hardly the walking thesaurus at the moment. I now look at other nurses I work with, some closeted and some openly gay, who never have any issues with their patients. I want to sit down to discuss their nursing practice and what I'm going through with this journal but it's hardly the conversation you have over morning tea.

The acceptance of course is not as wide amongst colleagues. Nursing is renowned for horizontal violence and what I have found in more than one instance is that if people have a problem with me in the workplace and are wanting to get even (especially in my role as manager) then they will use your sexuality to get maximum effect when driving the knife into your back.

I would like to see the day when I would feel comfortable as a male in nursing to be upfront and open about my sexuality in the workplace. I don't lie about my sexuality or my relationship these days but I guess I probably work at keeping things on a professional level to avoid discussion about my personal life. My partner, Jack, does not agree with this as he believes in being upfront about your sexuality, then if anybody begins to harass you about your sexuality you have a clear case of harassment. I prefer to live a more sedate and quiet life.

We also discussed staffing levels and protests against management in our discussion. I told Bev about how annoyed I was that in response to what people believe is short staffing they are not doing things for patients so that set goals are not achieved.

How do we get this point across to management/administration? I believe we meet them halfway. The ward where I am rostered is a surgical unit which is stuck in the 70s. When I first started in the hospital the patient ratio was one nurse to five patients. I spent most of my time wondering what to do with my spare time as the patients could only stand so much of my company. This was the case with most of the staff but most of them spent that time socialising at the desk. (I know I'm sounding like an old school charge nurse.)

My problem with this is that no patient care protocols have ever been developed, no education or orientation has ever been done and the only way to find things out is to ask the person in charge. None of this expertise is shared so that knowledge is power and you can make new staff feel inadequate for not knowing things.

A new Unit Manager was employed to try and change this and the changes to clinical pathways were enforced along with other changes and the staff have fought these changes all the way.

Gradually the unit will get there as they employ new younger staff who are developing patient care protocols as their expertise is developed. Where people like myself come into play at this point in time is to support the younger staff in their battles against the old school who still want to hold the power and prevent nurses having any autonomy and responsibility for their practice.

The greatest concern to me is that these poor kids are beaten around so badly when they make a mistake they are not learning. They are becoming defensive and with this I believe risk picking up all the bad habits from their peers.

An example of this was last evening when I was receiving handover from a young graduate who was looking after a patient newly diagnosed with a PE. I asked what the patient's O_2 saturation was and the grad told me she hadn't done it. I began to tell her why it would be a good idea to have done it and she began to get defensive. I then had to start again and say that I wasn't being critical, I was trying to help her understand what an important baseline observation this may be in this patient.

I look back over this journal and I think I'm beginning to sound like a very serious pain-in-the-arse type nurse. Not true.

Last night and tonight I have been working with Lea who typifies what I see as good nursing care. Lea takes the time to get to know every patient, gets the detailed life history. The patients want for nothing and feel free to ask any questions or for anything.

What I love about Lea is her story telling. She is one of those nurses who can keep you entertained for hours with the things she has seen and she paints every detail.

Earlier tonight we were talking of hospital training days and the dragon charge nurses we worked under.

Lea tells the story of her and two fellow students being based up in children's ward and asked what T's and A's were. Lea stood still and one nurse stood forward and said 'temperature', the other stood forward and said 'allergies'. They both had the crap blasted out of them. Now they repeat the scenario at every reunion.

It reminded me of Children's ward at my training hospital with the most bizarre charge nurse I have met in my nursing career. This charge nurse kept a running tally at the back of her writing pad of things that she would blast you for at the end of the day. My friend Judy and I were working together and when the charge nurse went to tea we did our usual and had a look to see what we had done wrong today. Judy had her usual list and under my name it had 'no complaints'. I stuck my chest out and thought I finally had it right. At the end of the day we were called in and Judy had the crap blasted out of her and I stood there thinking about 'no complaints' and wondering if I was actually going to be praised for my work.

The charge nurse finally turned to me and said that she noticed that I had written 'no complaints' on an obs chart. She then started yelling 'The child could be dead and making no complaints!' I thought Judy was going to wet herself. My big moment gone in one swoop.

Carol's stories

A story about ensuring effective care for a baby

On postnatal ward. Mother Jill Day 2, normal delivery. Strep B on vaginal swab. Baby obs—baby has slight temp, ?overwrapped, but also tachypnoea.

Most obs done Day 1 temp up slightly, slight tachypnoea.

Day 2 normal breathing but temp 37.5. In light of strep B, need for further consultation with RMO firstly and paediatrician if necessary.

RMO treatment ordered—MSU, chest X-ray and paediatric consultation.

I was not happy sitting on this baby so paediatrician was consulted and MSU, CXR, admission to SCN for observation.

Throughout discussed with Mum and Dad reasons for concern and possible reasons for temperature and complicating Strep B swab from mother.

Reflections

Covering my butt is smeared all through this event. How many times I did the temperature and respirations and then forcing (encouraging) the RMO to ring the paediatrician to make him aware of the situation and him ultimately responsible.

The role of the RMO was a time waster, it is the correct line of referral but if he didn't do what I wanted him to do I would not hesitate to go above their heads.

Explanations to the parents are my greatest assets. I can explain so they can understand, sometimes a bit verbosely but they got the message that it was a serious situation or at least could develop into one.

Did I push or over-treat on this baby? You can

never be too sure with a potential Strep B infection.
I was also conscious that a new student midwife
was taking over my patients and there was only one
midwife on the ward and she was also in charge.
    I am unaware if the baby was treated for Strep
B or just observed in SCN for awhile.

A critical friend's commentary and questions

In this story I detected Carol's anxiety about caring for a baby
at risk from streptococcal infection and her need to ensure that
the matter was investigated thoroughly.
    I offer these questions to Carol as a critical friend:

- Carol, what is missing from your account is how you felt
  about the situation. 'Reading between the lines' I infer that
  you were anxious for the wellbeing of the baby and for the
  parents, but you have not actually put yourself into the picture
  in other than a 'clinical' way. For example, you wrote about
  needing to cover your 'butt', the RMO as a time waster, and
  your concern that a 'new student midwife' was taking over
  your patients, yet you do not use words such as anxious,
  frustrated, worried, and so on. Look back over this story and
  insert words which tell me about how you were really feeling.

A story about a busy day

Normal Friday. Very busy antenatal clinic. I had six
patients and wow were they heavy.
    First patient had previous breakdown and was
presenting paranoid, anxious, disorganised. Patient
also aggressive. I talked for a long time with this
patient, normalising the baby's behaviour and discussing patient support systems—ECN, GP, social
worker, psychologist. I talked to her mother as well
to allow her to be in the situation.
    2. Caesarean section yesterday evening. Failed

induction for post dates. Oral pain relief and couldn't get baby to feed and no time for a bath. Patient's IDC out, IV capped. ED catheter removed, patient showered.

3. Caesarean section Day 3. I spent a few hours of back-breaking work to assist woman to breastfeed yesterday and today she gave up breastfeeding as it was too hard.

4. Premmie, 32 weeks with increased white cells in labour ward all day. Eventually delivered VBAC (vaginal birth after caesarean). Baby to SCN. I went to congratulate them at end of day.

5. Primip delivered during the night, assisted with breastfeed, no time for baby bath.

6. Caesarean section 2am, two-hourly PCA observations. Baby discharged from SCN. Temperature a bit low but when baby close to Mum temperature naturally came up to normal.

Reflections

A day allocated only six patients but they are more dependent and complicated than usual nursing patients.

One woman went to labour ward so I had five women and five babies. ?Ten patients.

Patient with psych history needed to be brought back to reality and referred. A number of hours' worth of counselling, discussing the observations of patients and their interaction with baby and this is included in the managed care plan for each client. This is indeed a case which needs further follow-up. This baby is 'at risk' and will eventually be referred to DOCS I think.

I felt exhausted both mentally and physically. I felt frustrated I couldn't give each parent my full attention.

There is a big pressure to 'finish work' in the morning but the old-fashioned hand-over and working together seems to be old thinking.

Solid breastfeeding assistance required along with Day 1 surgical patients and psychosomatic condition. One also had history of domestic violence. Wow. Now I am on holidays. Bye!!!!

A critical friend's commentary and questions

In this story Carol described a busy day just before she went on holidays.

I offer these questions to Carol as a critical friend:

- You wrote that you 'felt exhausted both mentally and physically' and frustrated that you could not give each parent your full attention. What constraints are operating in your workplace which prevent you from giving the care you would ideally choose to give?
- When you wrote about the 'old-fashioned hand-over and working together', were you saying that you miss these traditions and that they have useful purposes? What purposes did they serve? Why have these traditions gone? Are there any other strategies for ensuring that midwives work together?

As you can see, Carol writes in a short sentence style, but she still manages to pack a lot of information into her practice stories. Consider your commentary to Carol as her critical friend, in relation to pointing out what you see as possible practice approaches, issues and themes in her stories. If you go back to Chapter 4 you will see what Carol wrote about herself as she set out as a reflective practitioner. Look to see if there are connections with the content of Carols' practice stories and the ways she described herself as a child and a midwife.

SUMMARY

In this chapter I provided you with opportunities to read more practice stories from Esther, Michael and Carol, who shared their stories with you, as a means of improving your reflective skills and knowledge. I provided a commentary on their accounts and raised some questions as their critical friend. I also encouraged you to analyse their stories to locate their practice approaches, issues and themes, so that you could provide your commentary to them as a critical friend, and learn from their experiences.

11

Maintaining reflective practice

This chapter discusses maintaining your reflective practitioner mentality and the value of finding support systems to keep you on track. This may lead on to organising professional development seminars in your work setting in which to share your experiences or getting involved in research. In conclusion, this chapter and book end on a positive note as you contemplate the potential of embodying reflective practice in your everyday life and work.

AFFIRMING YOURSELF AS A REFLECTIVE PRACTITIONER

To become settled into your new life of reflection you may need to consider ways of affirming your intentions. The rites of passage from an unconsidered to a considered life are ways of affirming your new status. Among these rituals and symbols of transition are special forms of preparation and resolve that will buoy you up when you start to sink in the swell of daily responsibilities. In this section I suggest some ways of affirming yourself as a reflective practitioner, so that reflection becomes a daily habit based in pockets of silence; life in general becomes energised by seeing it freshly; and work remains interesting by staying alert to practice.

Creating a daily habit

To affirm your experience of reflection, it will be important to maintain your reflective practitioner mentality. It is easy to do something when it is novel. It is another thing to maintain something which has lost some of its initial appeal and requires a certain amount of discipline and attention for its continued use. Days of weakened resolve may come for you as a reflective practitioner.

Just as you wash and feed your body as part of your essential daily activities, it is also possible to find enough space in your day-to-day life for reflection. This does not necessarily mean that you will write in a journal or speak into an audiotape every workday, but it may mean that you will be engaged sufficiently in work as to reflect on it in some shape or form. In a practical sense, this may mean that you will use opportunities to take time out from the busyness of life to spend time in quietness.

Silence is the generative home of possibilities. Take time each day to find it, because it will not come to you unless you think it is important enough to seek it actively by doing nothing. It may seem like a contradiction to be active doing nothing, but unless you realise that silence is to be claimed, it will continue to elude you. Doing this and that can overtake life, so that your body rarely experiences immobility, silence and time for reflective thought. Consider the key activities of your day—simple things like washing, eating and socialising—and be alert to opportunities to be quiet, to go within and to 'just be' in the moment. From this place of quietness comes the potential for deep and effortless thought that springs up from a source of creativity and gives you clues and answers to puzzles that reside within you.

Seeing things freshly

Adopting a new way of seeing the events of everyday life can assist in affirming yourself as a reflective practitioner. This may mean that you try actively to keep a fresh perspective on ordinary aspects of life that you would otherwise have taken for granted. For example, what do you see when you open your eyes each morning? Have you ever really looked around the room, noticing its details? Have you ever looked carefully out the window and noticed the colours and moods of morning? As you step into active involvement in the day, start to be aware of all the little details of your life and the people with whom you interact. If these entities and people become a source of interest instead of familiarity, you may see them freshly, with new significance and potential for what and who they are and how they fit into the schemes and patterns of daily life.

Seeing the details of your life freshly will create a sense of constant connection and interest in your relationships to people and your environment. This will be excellent practice for the attentiveness you need as a reflective practitioner. For me, seeing things freshly is possible because I look out at the world from a fairly settled state inside myself, which allows me to focus on details and to be present. This way of seeing is gentle and quiet with wide eyes of interest. It is not busy and bustling with peering eyes of inquisitiveness. My advice is that you nurture a way of seeing from a quiet and steady state which allows you to look around like a tourist visiting a foreign country for the first time. You may learn to see things freshly each day, discriminating between accepting and contesting, and making sense in general of more and more aspects of your life.

Staying alert to practice

The need for seeing freshly in your personal life applies equally to your work life. You can affirm your status as a reflective practitioner by staying alert to your practice. Although you need to have a degree of comfort and familiarity with your work setting so you don't 'become a nervous wreck', too much familiarity can blind you to what is around you. You need to stay alert to notice the details that can keep you entrenched in unexamined clinical procedures, patterns of human relating and power plays. The point I am making is that work realities are complex and challenging, containing issues that relate to the need for ever-increasing technical knowledge, refinements of relationships, and a constant critique of power within the organisation in which you work. These issues present an immense challenge to stay alert to practice to monitor the moves and shifts in its nature and effects.

How do you stay alert on your shift? You cannot always predict how a shift at work may transpire. Sometimes it may be fast and action-packed and sometimes it may be slow and relatively uneventful. The point to consider is that the degree of busyness will not necessarily dictate your alertness. Yes, if you are busy you are attentive to what you are doing and how you are doing it, but you may not necessarily be alert to the fine details of interactions and outcomes. This state of alertness comes when you make conscious attempts to tune in as you work. You have to be 'at the controls' and not cruising through the challenges on autopilot. Conversely, you may not be alert just because you have more time on a quiet shift. This may be the very time at which you go into a holding pattern and fail to see the fine aspects of work because it is 'uneventful'. The quiet shifts may be your richest times of reflection, in terms of being alert to the taken-for-granted ways of thinking, doing, and being. In short, every moment of practice is a potential source of reflection, so stay alert to these opportunities.

FINDING SUPPORT SYSTEMS

Maintaining reflection will not be easy. I have seen people with the best intentions—including myself—throw reflective habits away when life overtakes them. I've made many resolutions over the years about what I intend to do for all kinds of aspects in my life, but I've since realised that I was actually hoping for ideal circumstances to see these resolutions take form. Life seldom runs to plan and many unforseen obstructions and challenges can get in the way of ideal circumstances. I imagine that when you resolve to maintain reflective processes, the trials of life will get in your way and your resolutions may not come to fruition. If this occurs, don't give in and 'throw the baby away with the bath water'. I've learned that the best way to keep a resolution alive is to hold on to the principle of the idea, even when the fine detail of my intentions go into recess.

Although your first step will be to affirm yourself as a reflective practitioner, by making reflection a daily habit, and taking measures to see life freshly and stay alert to practice, you will also benefit from support systems external to yourself. Even if you get underway with relative ease and confidence, you will also benefit from the support of other people who are practising reflection within the organisation and across disciplines.

Try to ascertain whether there are other clinicians engaged in reflective practice. You may find that there are 'closet' reflective practitioners inside your ward or unit, hospital or health region. People begin reflection through many sources, such as tertiary study, professional development courses, organisational seminars and so on. To find these people, you may need to leave a message pinned on a staff notice board, indicating that you are trying to begin a support group for reflective practitioners. You could suggest a meeting time, place and agenda and leave your contact details for the RSVP. You may be surprised who emerges out of the system.

Alternatively, you could send out an invitation on email within your organisation, or on the Internet, to access people more broadly, and set up electronic connections with other reflective practitioners. Check the listings already in use and you may find that you could join an established group within nursing and midwifery, or across health care professions and other disciplines such as education.

SHARING REFLECTION

Why not share reflective experiences in your ward, department or organisation, by organising a professional development seminar or conference? There are many possibilities. You could focus on nurses and midwives and/or other health workers, locally, nationally or internationally. I suggest that you start locally and within manageable proportions in your unit or hospital.

If you decide to organise a seminar, here is a checklist of details to consider as you plan for the event:

- *venue*—is it suitable and available?
- *program*—who will speak/present, for how long?
- *catering*—papers—will you provide participants with copies?
- *promotion*—how will you invite attendance?
- *sponsorship*—will you need to seek financial assistance?
- *equipment*—will speakers need audiovisual aids?
- *administration*—do you need a mechanism to budget and monitor numbers and costs?

Getting involved in research

Reflective processes work well in research projects, because the thinking required for research is similar to that required in maintaining reflective practice. In fact, in a research book of which I was co-author, this is the very tack I took to explain how to do qualitative research (Roberts and Taylor 1998). Knowledge, research, thinking and reflection are related through the ways they engage people in cognitive processes.

There is wide scope for research incorporating reflective processes or centred on experiences of reflective practice. For example, you could use reflective processes as a method for data collection in the field notes of a journal, or you could construct a research proposal focused on the nature and effects of reflective practice in any work context. You could undertake research in your work setting at any level, such as a ward, department or organisation. The project could involve nurses and midwives and other health workers. It could be planned to have a local, national or international focus and participation, depending on your knowledge and skills in establishing and maintaining research.

I cannot possibly hope to convey to you here all the information you need to do research. This has been the subject of many other books, some of which I will list now as good, practical approaches to doing research: Crookes and Davies (1998); LoBiondo and Haber (1994); Roberts and Taylor (1998). All I offer at this point are suggestions for research approaches to suit various kinds of reflection. It will be up to you to follow through and institute research projects according to your practice interests, and your knowledge and skill in undertaking research.

The basic reason for doing research is to find, explore and prove the worthiness of knowledge. Two words are inescapable in understanding how knowledge is generated: epistemology and ontology. *Epistemology* is the study of knowledge and how it is judged to be 'true'. I have placed inverted commas around the word true, because what truth is, and how it is generated and proven, will always be a source of debate. *Ontology* is the study of existence itself. Questions of human knowing and existing have been posed for ages through philosophical thought. Nurses and midwives are thinking workers, who need to ask questions about knowing and existing, because the answers to such questions form the substance of their disciplines.

The two main streams of inquiry are quantitative and qualitative. Quantitative research is also known as the empirico-analytical approach. It is based on 'the scientific

243

method', which stresses the attainment of rigour through the reliability and validity of projects, by using observational and analytic means to control and manipulate variables, to produce objective data that can be quantified to demonstrate the degree of statistical significance in cause and effect relationships. Technical reflection is best suited to quantitative research projects, although it can also be used in projects which mix quantitative and qualitative approaches.

Qualitative research attempts to explore the changing nature of knowledge, centred in the places, times and conditions in which people find themselves. There are many ways of categorising qualitative research; however, it is useful to think of qualitative categories as either interpretive or critical. Interpretive research approaches, such as grounded theory, phenomenology, ethnography and historical research, aim to create description and make sense of human phenomena and experiences. These approaches are best suited to practical reflection. Critical research methods of inquiry, such as action research, critical ethnography and feminist processes, are concerned mainly with social critique and change. These approaches arc best suited to emancipatory reflection.

The forms of reflection can be used as data collection methods in research projects. For example, a project examining the effectiveness of a clinical procedure could use technical reflective processes to facilitate critical thinking and problem-solving. The information gained through individual or collective discussions using objective argumentation is data. These processes could be used alone or in combination with other quantitative methods, such as experiments and structured observation. Research participants could keep reflective journals or use the questions posed by technical reflection as a stimulus for group discussion. The aim of research using technical reflection would be to satisfy the need for rational adaptations to work procedures and to maintain evidence-based practice.

Practical reflection may be used in any project which intends to explore the meaning of phenomena in nursing and midwifery. For example, a project may explore the meaning of illness as it is experienced. In this case, practical reflection could be encouraged in research participants by asking them to tell a story about the experience of their illness. The questions posed in the reflective process could facilitate the telling of the story to ensure that a rich description is achieved. Alternatively, the researcher or research team could keep reflective logs about their experiences of providing care for people.

Emancipatory reflection fits well with critical research, which aims to expose power relations and change the dominant forces constraining nurses' and midwives' practice. For example, a group of nurses or midwives could form an action research group and work collaboratively to bring about changes in their practice according to what matters most to themselves. This might mean that each person keeps a reflective log, parts of which are shared in the group to assist in deciding on the direction of the project. The group would work together to assess clinical problems and to suggest and trial strategies for change.

EMBODYING REFLECTIVE PRACTICE

As time passes, reflective practice will become a part of your life, so that it is in your daily repertoire. Just as you attend to the daily routines of life, so you will embody reflective practice, so that it becomes part of who and how you are. This may not mean that you remember to write in your journal or speak into an audiotape as a matter of daily routine, but it does mean that you do not lose your motivation to think reflectively and to be aware of the potential of making sense out of everyday events. You will remain aware of how life is constructed at home and work and why it might be so, and how it might be otherwise.

Your biggest challenge will be to remain aware of the danger of familiarity and the tendency to accept a given reality as though it is as it should be and could be no other way. Life will be seen as 'work in progress' in which nothing is perfect or complete and everything can be seen afresh constantly to reveal new insights and possibilities for interpretation and adaptation. Your personal growth as a person and health professional will continue as you open yourself up to the value of your own reflections and those gained in collaboration with your colleagues. This is not to imply that life will 'be upwards and onwards' without a hitch, but you will be actively and consciously aware of the events which used to pass you by, and you will have some processes whereby you can make sense of them.

SUMMARY

In this chapter I suggested that if you have found reflective processes useful for your work and life, you might like to consider letting other people know about them. To this end, I discussed the value of maintaining your reflective practitioner mentality and finding support systems to keep you on track. I described ways of organising professional development seminars in your work setting in which to share your experiences, and of getting involved in research. In conclusion, this chapter and book ended on a positive note as you contemplated the potential of embodying reflective practice in your everyday life and work. I wish you well.

References

Abdellah, F.G., Beland, I.L., Martin, A. and Matheney, R.V. 1960 *Patient-Centered Approaches to Nursing* Macmillan, New York

Allen, D., Benner P., Diekelmann N.L. 1986 Three paradigms for nursing research: Methodological implications, in P.L. Chinn (ed.) *Nursing Research Methodology: Issues And Implementation* Aspen, Rockville

Anderson, J.M. 1981 An interpretive approach to clinical nursing research *Nursing Papers* vol. 13 no. 4 pp. 6–12

——1987 Cultural context of caring *Canadian Critical Care Nursing* vol. 4 no. 4 pp. 7–13

——(ed.) 1996 *Thinking Management: Contemporary Approaches For Nurse Managers* Ausmed Publications, Melbourne

Bandman, E.L. and Bandman, B. 1995 *Critical Thinking in Nursing* 2nd edn Appleton and Lange, Norwalk

Baudrillard, J. 1988 *Selected Writings* Poster, M. (ed.) Stanford University Press, Stanford, Cal.

Belenky, M., Clinchy, B., Goldberger, N. and Tarule, J. 1986 *Women's Ways of Knowing* Basic Books, New York

Benner, P. 1984 *From Novice to Expert: Uncovering the Knowledge Embedded in Clinical Practice* Addison-Wesley, Menlo Park

Benner, P. and Tanner, C. 1987 Clinical judgement: How expert nurses use intuition *American Journal of Nursing* vol. 87 no. 23

Benner, P. and Wrubel, J. 1989 *The Primacy of Caring: Stress and Coping in Health and Illness* Addison-Wesley, Menlo Park

Bernstein, R.J. 1978 *The Restructuring of Social and Political Theory* University of Pennsylvania Press, Philadelphia

Boud, D. Keogh, R. and Walker, D. 1985 *Reflection: Turning Experience into Learning* Kagan, London

Boyd, E.M. and Fales, A.W. 1983 Reflective learning: Key to learning from experience *Journal of Humanistic Psychology* vol. 23 no. 2 pp. 99–117

Brennan, B.A. 1987 *Hands of Light: A Guide to Healing Through the Human Energy Field* Bantam Books, Toronto

——1993 *Light Emerging: The Journey of Personal Healing* Bantam Books, New York

Brown, S. and Lumley, J. 1994 Satisfaction with care in labour and birth: A survey of 790 Australian women *Birth* vol. 12 pp. 4–13

Caffarella, R. and Barnett, B. 1994 Characteristics of adult learners and foundations of experiential learning *New Directions for Adult and Continuing Education* no. 62 Summer Jossey Bass, San Francisco

Capra, F. 1988 *Uncommon Wisdom: Conversations with Remarkable People* Flamingo, London

——1992 *Belonging to the Universe: New Thinking about God and Nature* Penguin Books, London

Carper, B.A. 1978 Fundamental patterns of knowing in nursing *Advances in Nursing Science* vol. 1 pp. 13–23

Carr, W. and Kemmis, S. 1984 *Becoming Critical: Knowing Through Action Research* Deakin University Press, Victoria

Chinn, P.L. and Jacobs, M.K. 1983 *The Emergence of Nursing Theory* Mosby, St Louis

Chinn, P.L. and Kramer, M.K. 1991 *Theory and Nursing: A Systematic Approach* 3rd edn Mosby, St Louis

Clarke, B., James, C. and Kelly, J. 1996 Reflective practice: Reviewing the issues and refocussing the debate *International Journal of Nursing Studies* vol. 33 no. 2 pp. 191–9

Clinton, M. 1998 On reflection in action: Unaddressed issues in refocussing the debate on reflective practice *International Journal of Nursing Practice* vol. 4 no. 3 pp. 197–202

Conference 1990a *Nursing in the Nineties, RCNA 12th National Conference*, Sydney, May

Conference 1990b *Embodiment, Empowerment, Emancipation Conference*, Melbourne, February

Conference 1990c *Myth, Mystery and Metaphor*, 4th Nurse Education Conference proceedings, Melbourne, September

Conference 1991 *Science, Reflectivity and Nursing Care: Exploring the Dialectic*, Melbourne, arranged by The Dept of Nursing, La Trobe University, December

Conference 1992a *Nursing Kaleidoscope: Sharpen the Focus*, First National Nursing Forum, Adelaide, June

Conference 1992b: *The Postmodern Body: Health, Nursing and Narra-*

tive, Arranged by Departments of English and Nursing, La Trobe University, June

Conference 1992c *Nursing Research: Scholarship for Practice*, Research Conference, Deakin University, 1–2 July

Conference 1992d *Today's Education Formula: Tomorrow's Nursing Practice*, Faculty of Nursing, University of Sydney, 6–9 October

Conference 1993a *Critical Theory, Feminism and Nursing: Empowering Nursing's Future* arranged by the Department of Nursing, La Trobe University, Melbourne, 18–19 February

Conference 1993b: *Nursing Research: Scholarship for Practice*, Research Conference, Deakin University 8–9 July

Conway, J. 1994 Reflection, the art and science of nursing and the theory–practice gap *British Journal of Nursing* vol. 393 pp. 114–18

Couves, J. 1995 Working in practice in L. Page (ed.) *Effective Group Practice in Midwifery: Working with Women* Blackwell Science, Oxford

Cox, H., Hickson, P. and Taylor, B.J. 1991 Exploring reflection: Knowing and constructing the practice of nursing in G. Gray and R. Pratt (eds) *Towards a Discipline of Nursing* Churchill Livingstone, Melbourne, pp. 373–89

Crookes, P.A. and Davies, S. 1998 *Research into Practice* Balliere Tindall, Edinburgh

Crowder, E.L.M. 1985 Historical perspectives of nursing's professionalism *Occupational Health Nursing* vol. 33 no. 4 pp. 184–90

Cunningham, J. 1993 Experiences of Australian mothers who gave birth either at home, at a birth centre, or in hospital labour wards *Social Science of Medicine* vol. 36 no. 4 pp. 475–83

Dilthey, W. 1985 *Poetry and Experience: Selected Works vol. V* Princeton University Press, New Jersey

Duffy, E. 1995 Horizontal violence: A conundrum for nursing *Collegian* vol. 2 no. 2 pp. 5–17

Dunlop. M. 1986 Is a science of caring possible? *Journal of Advanced Nursing*, vol. 11 pp. 661–70

——1988 Science and caring: Are they compatible? *Shaping Nursing Theory And Practice: The Australian Context*, Lincoln School of Health Sciences, Department of Nursing, LaTrobe University, Melbourne

——1986 Is a science of caring possible? *Journal of Advanced Nursing*, vol. 11 pp. 661–70

Easwaren, E. 1990 *The Bhagavad Gita* Nilgiri Press, California

Ehrenreich, B. and English, D. 1973 *Witches Midwives and Nurses: A History of Women Healers* Writers and Readers Publishing Cooperative, London

Eliade, M. and Couliano, I.P. 1991 *The Eliade Guide to World Religions* Harper, San Francisco

Executive Summary 1994 *Nursing Education in Australian Universities: Report of the National Review of Nurse Education in the Higher Education Sector 1994 and Beyond* Australian Government Publishing Service, Canberra

Fay, B. 1975 *Social Theory and Political Practice* George Allen & Unwin, London

——1987 *Critical Social Science: Liberation and Its Limits* Polity Press, Cambridge

——1988 *Social Theory and Political Practice* George Allen & Unwin Ltd, London

Frederick, H. and Northam, E. 1938 *A Textbook of Nursing Practice* Macmillan, New York

Freidson, E. 1970 *Profession of Medicine A Study of the Sociology of Applied Knowledge* Harper and Row, New York

Gadamer, H-G. 1975 *Truth and Method* in G. Barden and J. Cumming (eds) and trans, Seabury, New York

Giroux, H.A. 1983 *Theory and Resistance in Education: A Pedagaogy for the Opposition* Bergin and Garvey, Massachusetts

——1990 *Curriculum Discourse as Postmodernist Critical Practice* Deakin University Press, Geelong

Glass, N. 1997 Horizontal violence in nursing *The Australian Journal of Holistic Nursing* vol. 4 no. 1 pp. 15–21

Gray, G. and Pratt, R. (eds) 1991 *Toward a Discipline of Nursing* Churchill Livingstone, Melbourne

Greenwood, J. 1993 Reflective practice: A critique of the work of Argyris and Schön *Journal of Advanced Nursing* vol. 18 pp. 1183–7

——(ed.) 1996 *Nursing Theory in Australia: Development and Application* Harper Educational, Australia

Habermas, J. 1972 *Knowledge and Human Interests* Heinemann, London

Heidegger, M. 1962 *Being and Time* in J. Macquarrie and E. Robinson (trans) Harper and Row, New York

Henderson, V. 1955 *Textbook of Principles and Practice of Nursing* Macmillan, New York

Hickson, P. 1991 The promises of critical theory, paper presented at the *Embodiment, Empowerment, Emancipation Conference*, Melbourne, February, 1990 in NPR806 Study Guide, Deakin University, Geelong

Holmes, C. 1990 Alternatives to natural science foundations for nursing *International Journal of Nursing Studies* vol. 27 no. 3 pp. 187–98

——1992 The drama of nursing *Journal of Advanced Nursing* vol. 17 pp. 954–60

Houston, J. 1987 *The Search for the Beloved: Journeys in Sacred Psychology* Crucible, California

Hoy, W.K. and Miskel, C.G. 1982 *Educational Administration—Theory, Research and Practice* Random House, New York

Johns, C. and Freshwater, D. 1998 *Transforming Nursing Through Reflective Practice* Blackwell Science, Oxford

Judith, A. 1992 *Wheels of Life: A User's Guide to the Chakra System* Llewellyn Publications, St Paul, Minnesota

Keleher, H. and McInerney, F. (eds) 1998 *Nursing Matters: Critical Sociological Perspectives* Churchill Livingstone, Australia

Kelly, K. 1985 Nurse practitioner challenges to the orthodox structure of health care delivery: Regulation and restraints on trade *American Journal of Law and Medicine* vol. 11 no. 2 pp. 195–225

Kermode, S. 1994 The organisation: A problem for the professionalisation of nursing *Contemporary Nurse* vol. 3 no. 3 pp. 110–17

Kermode, S. and Brown, C. 1996 The postmodernist hoax and its effects on nursing *The International Journal of Nursing Studies* vol. 31 no. 4 pp. 1–10

Kestenbaum, V. 1982 (ed.) *The Humanity of the Ill: Phenomenological Perspective* University of Tennessee Press, Knoxville

King, I.M. 1971 *Toward a Theory for Nursing: General Concepts of Human Behaviour* John Wiley, New York

Kinlein, M.L. 1977 *Independent Nursing Practice with Clients* Lippincott, Philadelphia

Kitzinger, S. 1991 Why women need midwives in S. Kitzinger (ed.) *The Midwife Challenge* Pandora, London

Kretlow, F. 1989–1990 A phenomenological view of illness *The Australian Journal of Advanced Nursing* vol. 7 no. 2 pp. 8–10

Lawler, J. 1991 *Behind the Screens: Nursing, Somology and the Problem of The Body* Churchill-Livingstone, Melbourne

Leininger, M. 1985 *Qualitative Research Methods in Nursing* Grune and Stratton, New York

LoBiondo G. and Haber J. 1994 *Nursing Research: Methods, Critical Appraisal, and Utilisation* Mosby, St Louis

Lumby, J. 1991 *Nursing: Reflecting on an Evolving Practice* Deakin University Press, Geelong

Maslow, A.H. 1970 *Motivation and Personality* Harper and Row, New York

McCool, W. and McCool, S. 1989 Feminism and nurse-midwifery: Historical overview and current issues *Journal of Nurse-Midwifery* vol. 345 no. 6, pp. 323–34

McMahon, R. and Pearson, A. (eds) 1991 *Nursing as Therapy* Chapman and Hall, London

Merton, R.K. 1957 Continuities in the theory of reference groups and social structure *Social Theory and Social Structure* The Free Press, New York

Mezirow, J. 1981 A critical theory of adult learning and education *Adult Education* vol. 32 no. 1 pp. 3–24

Munhall, P. and Oiler, C.J. (eds) 1986 *Nursing Research: A Qualitative Perspective* Appleton-Century-Crofts, Norwalk

Newell, R. 1992 Anxiety, accuracy and reflection: The limits of professional development *Journal of Advanced Nursing* vol. 17 pp. 1326–33

Nightingale, F. 1893 in L. Seymer (comp.) *Selected Writings of Florence Nightingale* 1955 Macmillan, New York

Oakley, A. and Houd, S. 1990 *Helpers in Childbirth: Midwifery Today* Hemisphere Publishing, USA

Oiler, C. 1982 The phenomenological approach in nursing research *Nursing Research* vol. 31 no. 3 pp. 171–81

——1986 Phenomenology: the method in P. Munhall and C.J. Oiler (eds) *Nursing Research: A Qualitative Perspective* Appleton-Century-Crofts, Norwalk

Orem, D. 1959 *Guides for Developing Curricula for the Education of Practical Nurses* Government Printing Office, Washington, DC

Orlando, I.J. 1961 *The Dynamic Nurse–Patient Relationship* Putnam's, New York

Parker, J.M. 1988 Theoretical perspectives in nursing: From microphysics to hermeneutics *Third Nursing Research Forum* Lincoln School of Health Sciences, La Trobe University, Melbourne

Parse, R.R. 1985 *Nursing Research: Qualitative Methods* Brady, Bowie US

——1987 *Nursing Science: Major Paradigms Theories and Critiques* W.B. Saunders, Philadelphia

Paterson, J. and Zderad, L. 1976 *Humanistic Nursing* Wiley, New York

Pearson, A. 1988 (ed.) *Primary Nursing* Croom Helm, London

——1989 Translating rhetoric into practice: Theory in action *National Nursing Theory Conference*, School of Nursing Studies, Sturt, South Australian College of Advanced Education

Pearson, A., Borbasi S., Fitzgerald M., Kowanko I. and Walsh K. 1997 Evidence based nursing: An examination of nursing within the international evidence based health care practice movement RCNA Discussion Document no. 1 *Nursing Review* Sydney

Peplau, H.E. 1952 *Interpersonal Relations in Nursing* Putnam, New York

Polgar, S. and Thomas, S.A. 1995 *Introduction to Research in the Health Sciences* 3rd edn Churchill Livingstone, Melbourne

Polit, D.F. and Hungler, B.P. 1997 *Essentials of Nursing Research: Methods, Appraisal and Utilization* Lippincott, Philadelphia

Roberts, K. and Taylor, B. 1998 *Nursing Research Processes: An Australian Perspective* Nelson ITP, Melbourne

Robinson, D. 1978 *Patients, Practitioners and Medical Care: Aspects of*

Medical Sociology William Heinemann Medical Books, Great Britain

Rogers, M. 1961 *Educational Revolution in Nursing* Macmillan, New York

Rothwell, H. 1996 Changing childbirth—changing nothing *Midwives* vol. 109 no. 1306 pp. 291–4

Roy, C. 1976 *Introduction to Nursing: An Adaptation Model* Prentice-Hall, Englewood Cliffs

Schön, D.A. 1983 *The Reflective Practitioner: How Practitioners Think in Action* Basic Books, New York

——1987 *Educating the Reflective Practitioner Towards a New Design for Teaching and Learning in the Professions* Jossey Bass, San Francisco

Seldes, G. 1983 *The Great Quotations* The Citadel Press, New Jersey

Short, S.D. and Sharman, E. 1987 The nursing struggle in Australia, *Image: Journal of Nursing Scholarship* vol. 19 no. 4 pp. 197–200

Shorten, A. and Wallace, M. 1997 Evidence based practice: The future is clear *Australian Nursing Journal* vol. 4 no. 6 pp. 22–4

Smyth, W.J. 1986a *Reflection-in-action EED432 Educational Leadership in Schools* Deakin University Geelong

——1986b The reflective practitoner in nursing education Unpublished paper to the Second National Nursing Education Seminar, SACAE, Adelaide

Speake, J. (ed.) 1991 *A Treasury of Biblical Quotations* Ivy Leaf, London

Speedy, S. 1987 Feminism and the professionalization of nursing *The Australian Journal of Advanced Nursing*, vol. 4 no. 2 pp. 20–8

——1988 Feminism and nursing: Theory to practice *Shaping Nursing Theory and Practice: The Australian Context* Department of Nursing, LaTrobe University, Melbourne

Stein, L. 1967 The doctor–nurse game in R. Dingwall and J. McIntosh (eds) *Readings in the Sociology of Nursing* Churchill Livingstone, Edinburgh

Stone, W. 1987 *Poems of Henry Lawson* Landsdowne Press, Sydney

Street, A. 1990 *Nursing Practice: High Hard Ground Messy Swamps and the Pathways in Between* Deakin University Press, Geelong

——1991 *From Image to Action: Reflection in Nursing Practice* Deakin University Press, Geelong

——1992 *Inside Nursing: A Critical Ethnography of Clinical Nursing* SUNY, New York

——1995 *Nursing Replay: Researching Nursing Culture Together* Churchill Livingstone, Melbourne

Sullivan, D. and Weitz, R. 1998 *Labour Pains: Modern Midwifery and Homebirth* Yale University Press, New Haven

Taylor, B.J. 1992 From helper to human: A reconceptualisation of the nurse as person *Journal of Advanced Nursing* vol. 17 pp. 1042–9

——1994 *Being Human: Ordinariness in Nursing* Churchill Livingstone, Melbourne

——1997 Big battles for small gains: A cautionary note for teaching reflective processes in nursing and midwifery *Nursing Inquiry* vol. 4 pp. 19–26

——1998, Locating a phenomenological perspective of reflective nursing and midwifery practice by contrasting interpretive and critical reflection in C. Johns and D. Freshwater (eds) *Transforming Nursing Through Reflective Practice* Blackwell Science, Oxford, pp. 134–50

Taylor, B., King, V. and Stewart, J. 1995 Reflective midwifery practice: Facilitating midwives' practice insights using a distance education reflective practitioner model *International Journal of Nursing Practice*, vol. 1 no. 1 pp. 26–31

Tellis Nayak, M. and Tellis Nayak, V. 1984 Games that professionals play: The social psychology of physician–nurse interaction, *Social Science and Medicine*, vol. 18 no. 12 pp. 1063–9

The Illustrated Stratford Shakespeare 1982 Chancellor Press, London

The Concise English Dictionary 1984 Omega Books, London

Travelbee, J. 1971 *Interpersonal Aspects of Nursing* in F.A. Davis, Philadelphia

van Hooft, S., Gillam, L. and Byrnes, M., 1995 *Facts and Values: An Introduction to Critical Thinking for Nurses* Maclennan and Petty, Sydney

Watson, J. 1981 Nursing's scientific quest *Nursing Outlook* vol. 29 no. 7 pp. 413–16

——1985 *Nursing: Human Science and Human Care: A Theory of Nursing* Appleton-Century-Crofts, Norwalk

Webster, N. 1972 *The International Webster Encyclopedic Dictionary* Tabor House, New York

Wiedenbach, E. 1964 *Clinical Nursing: A Helping Art* Springer Publishing, New York

Wilkinson, J.M. 1996 *Nursing Process: A Critical Thinking Approach* Addison-Wesley Nursing, Menlo Park, Cal.

World Health Organisation 1985 *Having a Baby in Europe: Report on a Study* World Health Organisation, Copenhagen

Index